Pharmacokinetic and Pharmacodynamic Drug Interactions Associated with Antiretroviral Drugs

Tony K.L. Kiang • Kyle John Wilby
Mary H.H. Ensom
Editors

Pharmacokinetic and Pharmacodynamic Drug Interactions Associated with Antiretroviral Drugs

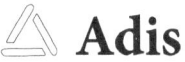 Adis

Editors
Tony K.L. Kiang
Faculty of Pharmaceutical Sciences
The University of British Columbia
Vancouver
BC
Canada

Mary H.H. Ensom
Faculty of Pharmaceutical Sciences
The University of British Columbia
Vancouver
BC
Canada

Kyle John Wilby
College of Pharmacy
Qatar University
Doha
Qatar

ISBN 978-981-10-9530-6   ISBN 978-981-10-2113-8   (eBook)
DOI 10.1007/978-981-10-2113-8

Printed on acid-free paper

This Adis imprint is published by Springer Nature
The registered company is Springer Science+Business Media Singapore Pte Ltd.
The registered company address is: 152 Beach Road, #22-06/08 Gateway East Singapore 189721, Singapore

Acknowledgment

We thank Samuel E. Gilchrist, Ph.D. sam_gilchrist@me.com for creating Fig. 1.1 specifically for this book.

Contents

Chapter 1
Introduction

Kyle John Wilby, Tony K.L. Kiang, and Mary H.H. Ensom

The advent of HIV and the related acquired immune deficiency syndrome (AIDS) was one of the most significant medical and public health findings of modern times [1]. It is arguable that no other disease has had as great of an impact on all aspects of society, including social, political, health, education, and legal systems worldwide. Its devastating impact on developing countries in Africa has led to increases in child morbidity and mortality, as well as a higher prevalence of orphaned children due to its effect on adult populations [2]. Economically, it has changed the way countries perceive treatment benefits and funding for harm reduction strategies [3].

Throughout the last three decades, the pharmaceutical industry has produced highly effective antiretroviral medications that significantly prolong life and reduce virus transmission [4]. Although no cure exists, these medications suppress the virus to undetectable levels and patients can live long, healthy lives if strictly adherent to treatment regimens. This is generally true for patients living in developed regions, as there are minimal barriers to drug access and knowledgeable care providers. However, access to care remains a major barrier for those living in many countries and those countries with developing healthcare systems [5].

K.J. Wilby
College of Pharmacy, Qatar University, Doha, Qatar
e-mail: kjw@qu.edu.qa

T.K.L. Kiang • M.H.H. Ensom (✉)
Faculty of Pharmaceutical Sciences,
The University of British Columbia,
Vancouver, BC, Canada
e-mail: tkiang@gmail.com; mary.ensom@ubc.ca

© Springer Science+Business Media Singapore 2016   1
T.K.L. Kiang et al. (eds.), *Pharmacokinetic and Pharmacodynamic Drug Interactions Associated with Antiretroviral Drugs*,
DOI 10.1007/978-981-10-2113-8_1

1.1 HIV Virus Lifecycle

The lifecycle of HIV with associated targets for antiretroviral therapy is given in Fig. 1.1. The lifecycle can be described in seven distinct stages [6]. Stage 1 occurs after the HIV virus enters the body and *binds* (attaches) to the CD4 cell. The CCR5 antagonists work at this stage to inhibit entry of HIV into the cell. Stage 2 occurs when the HIV envelope and cell membrane of the CD4 cell *fuse* and allow for the virus to enter the cell. The fusion inhibitors work at this stage to block fusion between the virus and cell. Stage 3 occurs inside the CD4 cell where the virus uses *reverse transcription* to convert HIV RNA into HIV DNA. This allows for viral DNA to be combined with the cellular DNA at the nucleus level. Both nucleoside reverse-transcriptase inhibitors (NRTIs) and nonnucleoside reverse transcriptase inhibitors (NNRTIs) work at this stage to inhibit viral reverse transcriptase. Stage 4 occurs inside the CD4 cell nucleus where HIV integrase is released to *integrate* viral DNA into the DNA of the host cell. This stage is the target of integrase inhibitors. Stage 5

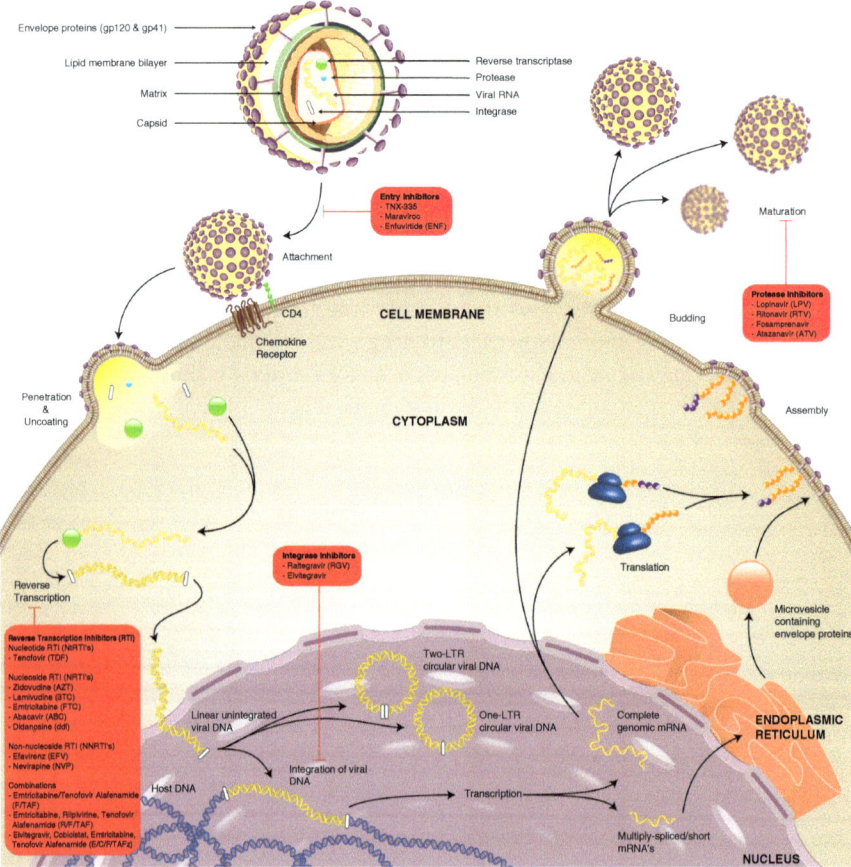

Fig. 1.1 Lifecycle of HIV with associated targets for antiretroviral therapy (This figure was created by Samuel E. Gilchrist, Ph.D. sam_gilchrist@me.com specifically for this book)

occurs when the HIV virus begins to *replicate* by using the CD4 cell to generate viral proteins. Stage 6 is based on the *assembly* of the new viral proteins with movement of the proteins and viral RNA to the surface of the cell. Stage 7 occurs when these newly formed noninfectious viruses *bud* from the cell and release protease to break the long immature chains into smaller HIV proteins that combine to form mature (infectious) HIV. Protease inhibitors work on this stage to prevent maturation of the virus [6].

1.2 Epidemiology

According to statistics from 2012, there were approximately 35.3 million people living with HIV worldwide [4]. The large majority (70.8%) of these infections were located in sub-Saharan Africa. Interestingly, the global prevalence has increased in recent years yet the annual incidence has decreased. This trend can be attributed to greater access to antiretroviral therapy that is allowing infected patients to live longer as well as to reductions in transmission. Decreased mother-to-child transmission has also been observed throughout the last decade (decrease of 38% between 2009 and 2012 in 21 priority African countries in the UN Programme on HIV/AIDS) [4]. However, the impact of HIV on society is still great. In 2010, it was the leading cause of disability-adjusted life years for people aged 30–44 years [4]. Mortality from AIDS is decreasing but still remains a major global health concern in underdeveloped nations.

1.3 Risk Factors

Risk factors for transmission of HIV are many and complex. The most important factor is deemed to be the viral load of the infected partner during sexual transmission. There appears to be a 2.4 times increased risk for every 1 log10 increase in viral RNA [7]. Other factors include existence of other sexually transmitted infections, pregnancy, and receptive anal intercourse. Male circumcision is associated with a reduced risk of transmission. Behavioral factors include having multiple sexual partners, injection and noninjection drug use, men who have sex with men, and commercial sex workers. Sex inequality and partner abuse may also be associated with increased transmission [4].

1.4 Diagnosis

All people with risk factors for HIV transmission should be encouraged to seek medical care for testing on a regular basis. Both point-of-care and laboratory testing methods are available [8]. Advantages of point-of-care testing are convenience and instant results for patients potentially lost to follow up. However, these tests are associated with a longer window period for HIV detection than traditional laboratory methods. If a positive result is obtained by point-of-care testing, a confirmatory laboratory test should be completed [8]. Additional tests to be ordered for positive patients include CD4 count, HIV viral load, and resistance testing [9]. These tests help inform treatment decisions as well as determine indications for opportunistic infection prophylaxis. CD4 counts and viral loads are also essential for monitoring of patients once they are established on therapy.

The Center for Disease Control recommends a laboratory testing algorithm for the diagnosis of HIV. The first stage of the algorithm is to conduct a test for HIV with an approved antigen/antibody combination immunoassay that detects both HIV-1 and HIV-2 antibodies as well as HIV-1 p24 antigen. If nonreactive, no further testing is required. If reactive, an immunoassay that differentiates between HIV-1 and HIV-2 should be completed. Specimens reactive on the initial antigen/antibody test but nonreactive or indeterminate on the differentiation immunoassay should be tested for HIV-1 nucleic acid. Testing abilities may vary depending on location of the laboratory and resources available [10].

1.5   Clinical Guidelines

The latest recommendations for initiating therapy state that antiretroviral therapy is recommended for all infected individuals, in order to reduce morbidity and mortality associated with infection and to prevent HIV transmission [9]. Therapy can be delayed depending on clinical and/or psychosocial factors but should be initiated as soon as possible. As such, education regarding adherence and the importance of therapy is required to optimize outcomes. These new recommendations differ from past recommendations that based treatment decisions on a target CD4 T-lymphocyte cell count threshold. This is primarily due to the results of two major studies that showed improved clinical outcomes with early or immediate initiation of antiretroviral therapy [11, 12].

Many drug classes are available to treat HIV and are discussed more comprehensively in Chap. 2. Nucleoside reverse transcriptase inhibitors (NRTIs) remain the cornerstone of therapy and are typically combined with at least one additional active agent from a different class. Nonnucleoside reverse transcriptase inhibitors (NNRTIs,), protease inhibitors (PIs), and integrase strand transfer inhibitors (INSTIs) remain active drugs with favorable efficacy and safety profiles [9]. Other drug classes (fusion and entry inhibitors) are also available for use.

Initial treatment of HIV consists of combinations of antiretroviral medications with differing mechanisms of action. Typically, a treatment-naïve patient will receive two NRTIs in combination with a third active agent. The third agent is generally chosen from the NNRTI, INSTI, or PI classes. Current first-line recommended regimens for treatment-naïve patients are given in Table 1.1. Briefly, INSTI and PI-based regimens are now considered preferable, based on both efficacy and safety profiles [9]. Alternative regimens are also available and given in Table 1.1. Selection of the most appropriate regimen is based on a number of factors that include organ function, preexisting medical conditions, pill burden, genotype, and patient preference. Treatment recommendations differ for special populations such as children,

Table 1.1 First-line and alternative regimens used for the treatment of HIV [9]

Priority	Core component	Agents
First-line regimens	Integrase inhibitor	Dolutegravir, abacavir, lamivudine
		Dolutegravir, tenofovir, emtricitabine
		Elvitegravir, cobicistat, tenofovir, emtricitabine
		Raltegravir, tenofovir, emtricitabine
	Protease inhibitor	Darunavir, ritonavir, tenofovir, emtricitabine
Alternative regimens	Nonnucleoside reverse transcriptase inhibitor	Efavirenz, tenofovir, emtricitabine Rilpivirine, tenofovir, emtricitabine
	Protease inhibitor	Atazanavir, tenofovir, emtricitabine
		Atazanavir, ritonavir, tenofovir, emtricitabine
		Darunavir, ritonavir, abacavir, lamivudine
		Darunavir, cobicistat, abacavir, lamivudine
		Darunavir, cobicistat, tenofovir, emtricitabine

pregnant women, and those patients with drug resistance. Guidelines and consensus statements are available to help guide decision making for these patients [9].

Many factors exist that may influence choice of first-line agents [9]. First, regimens with abacavir should be used only for patients who test negative for HLA-B*5701. The presence of this allele is associated with increased hypersensitivity to abacavir. Renal function in terms of creatinine clearance is important for initiation of tenofovir therapy, and thresholds must be checked before deciding on a specific formulation. Finally, viral load and CD4 count are important for initiation of rilpivirine therapy as this drug should be initiated only in patients with HIV RNA <100,000 copies per mL and CD4 count >200 cells/mm^3.

Special attention must be paid to adherence to antiretroviral therapy. Identified factors affecting adherence include untreated psychological disorders, neurocognitive impairment, active substance abuse, unstable housing, side effects, and lack of follow-up [9]. Clinicians should proactively attempt to recognize these factors and provide education, referral, and support when needed to assist patients in successfully adhering to therapy. Choice of regimen is also important for patient convenience [13].

1.6   Overview of Drug Interactions

Pharmacokinetic drug interactions occur when one agent leads to increases or decreases in exposure of another. These interactions occur during absorption, distribution, metabolism, or elimination of the affected drug [14]. Associated exposure changes may lead to decreased therapeutic effects (with decreased exposure) or increased effect/toxicity (with increased exposure). However, not all pharmacokinetic interactions will result in a change in clinical effect. This is dependent on many factors but primarily whether or not a dose- or concentration-effect relationship is present for the affected agent. Strategies such as therapeutic drug monitoring may help to overcome and monitor pharmacokinetic drug interactions when a concentration-effect relationship exists but only when benefit has clearly been established.

Pharmacodynamic drug interactions occur when the combination of drugs results in additive, synergistic, or antagonistic effects [14]. This largely occurs when drugs act at the same or similar receptor sites. These types of interactions may be related to efficacy and/or safety. For example, additive interactions may improve therapeutic efficacy or could result in increases of overlapping toxicity. The same may be said for synergistic interactions. Antagonistic interactions typically result in decreased drug activity and/or therapeutic effect. While these interactions are typically overshadowed by pharmacokinetic interactions, they must be monitored carefully to ensure patients achieve optimal efficacy and safety as part of the therapeutic regimen.

1.7 Summary

HIV is a changing disease yet still remains one of the greatest infectious disease health burdens to date. Fortunately, the advent of antiretroviral combinations and development of newer potent agents with less toxicity is allowing for increased survival of HIV patients. Due to the complexity of regimen combinations, however, patients are at great risk of experiencing pharmacokinetic and pharmacodynamic drug interactions. The following chapters will provide more background on HIV management and associated interactions.

References

1. Piot P, Bartos M, Ghys PD, Walker N, Schwartlander B (2001) The global impact of HIV/AIDS. Nature 410(6831):968–973
2. Foster G, Williamson J (2000) A review of current literature of the impact of HIV/AIDS on children in sub-Saharan Africa. AIDS 14(Suppl 3):S275–284
3. Dixon S, McDonald S, Roberts J (2002) The impact of HIV and AIDS on Africa's economic development. BMJ 324(7331):232–234B
4. Maartens G, Celum C, Lewin SR (2014) HIV infection: epidemiology, pathogenesis, treatment, and prevention. Lancet 384(9939):258–271
5. U.S. Department of Health & Human Services. Global Statistics. 2015. Available at https://www.aids.gov/hiv-aids-basics/hiv-aids-101/global-statistics/. Accessed 18 June 2016
6. AIDSinfo. HIV overview: the HIV lifecycle. Updated Sep 22, 2015. Available from: https://aidsinfo.nih.gov/education-materials/fact-sheets/19/73/the-hiv-life-cycle#. Accessed 14 June 2016.

7. Quinn TC, Wawer MJ, Sewankambo N, Serwadda D, Li C, Wabwire-Mangen F et al (2000) Viral load and heterosexual transmission of human immunodeficiency virus type 1: Rakai Project Study Group. N Eng J Med 342(13):921–929

8. Broeckaert L, Challacombe L. Rapid point-of-care HIV testing: a review of the evidence. Prevention in Focus 2015. Available from: http://www.catie.ca/en/pif/spring-2015/rapid-point-care-hiv-testing-review-evidence. Accessed 19 June 2016

9. Panel on Antiretroviral Guidelines for Adults and Adolescents. Guidelines for the use of anti-retroviral agents in HIV-1 infected adults and adolescents. Department of Health and Human Services. 2016. Available at http://www.aidsinfo.nih.gov/ContentFiles/AdultandAdolescentGL.pdf. Accessed 15 June 2016

10. Centers for Disease Control and Prevention (CDC) and Association of Public Health Laboratories. Laboratory testing for the diagnosis of HIV infection: updated recommendations. Published June 27, 2014. Available at http://dx.doi.org/10/15620/cdc.23447. Accessed 14 June 2016

11. INSIGHT START Study Group, Lundgren JD, Babiker AG, Gordin F, Emery S, Grund B et al (2015) Initiation of antiretroviral therapy in early asymptomatic HIV infection. N Engl J Med 373(9):795–807

12. TEMPRANO ANRS 12136 Study Group, Danel C, Moh R, Gabillard D, Badje A, Le Carrou J et al (2015) A trial of early antiretroviral and isoniazid preventive therapy in Africa. N Engl J Med 373(9):808–822

13. Trotta MP, Ammassari A, Melzi S, Zaccarelli M, Ladisa N, Sighinolfi L et al (2002) Treatment-related factors and highly active antiretroviral therapy adherence. J Acquir Immune Defic Syndr 31(Suppl 3):S128–S131

14. Palleria C, Di Paolo A, Giofre C, Caglioti C, Leuzzi G, Sinischalchi A et al (2013) Pharmacokinetic drug-drug interaction and their implication in clinical management. J Res Med Sci 18(7):601–610

Chapter 2
HIV-Associated Comorbidities

Kyle John Wilby, Tony K.L. Kiang, and Mary H.H. Ensom

Populations at higher risk of contracting HIV are typically prone to comorbidities that may increase the potential for actual and potential drug interactions with antiretrovirals [1]. These can include both infectious and noninfectious comorbidities. Interactions may be due to intrinsic pharmacokinetic properties of co-administered agents or their respective pharmacodynamic effects. A summary of common comorbidities with assessments of drug interaction potential is given below and presented in Table 2.1. These comorbidities are identified by clinical guidance documents published by the World Health Organization (WHO) [2]. Notably, HIV patients may also be at higher risk of other comorbidities (such as cardiovascular diseases and diabetes), but this is largely dependent on the specific context or population studied [3].

K.J. Wilby
College of Pharmacy, Qatar University, Doha, Qatar
e-mail: kjw@qu.edu.qa

T.K.L. Kiang • M.H.H. Ensom (✉)
Faculty of Pharmaceutical Sciences, The University of British Columbia,
Vancouver, BC, Canada
e-mail:tkiang@gmail.com; mary.ensom@ubc.ca

© Springer Science+Business Media Singapore 2016
T.K.L. Kiang et al. (eds.), *Pharmacokinetic and Pharmacodynamic Drug Interactions Associated with Antiretroviral Drugs*,
DOI 10.1007/978-981-10-2113-8_2

Table 2.1 Common comorbidities that increase potential for drug interactions in HIV-infected patients

Comorbidity	Interaction potential	Suggested actions
Tuberculosis	High	Modification of rifamycin therapy, where applicable
Malaria	Moderate	Careful monitoring of therapeutic outcomes associated with malaria
Hepatitis B and C	Moderate	Thorough assessment of overlapping toxicities associated with new direct acting antiviral regimens
Mental health disorders	Moderate	Choice of neuroactive agents to be least likely for interactions with antiretrovirals Careful monitoring of both efficacy and safety outcomes, especially for overlapping toxicities (QT prolongation, hepatotoxicity)

2.1   Tuberculosis

Tuberculosis is the most common life-threatening opportunistic infection in patients with HIV [4]. As such, patients with tuberculosis must be given prompt treatment, including concurrent antiretrovirals. Tuberculosis puts patients at greater risk of drug interactions due to complexity of treatment regimens and interaction potential of both antitubercular and antiretroviral drugs [2]. Drug regimens used to treat tuberculosis typically consist of four agents, namely rifampin, isoniazid, pyrazinamide, and ethambutol [5]. Each agent has a unique pharmacokinetic profile that increases potential for drug interactions as well as pharmacodynamic effects that could enhance toxicity and put patients at risk of harmful outcomes. Therefore, careful management of these patients must be undertaken to ensure therapy is not compromised for HIV or tuberculosis comorbidities and to ensure patient safety.

Some strategies have attempted to decrease drug interaction potential of first-line agents in recent years. Specifically, international guidelines currently recommend that rifabutin instead of rifampin be given to patients receiving protease inhibitors as part of their antiretroviral therapy [5]. This consideration is justified based on the decreased drug interaction potential of rifabutin versus rifampin with protease inhibitors [6]. It is also acceptable, but not mandatory, to use rifabutin in patients taking nonprotease inhibitor based regimens. It should be noted that the use of rifapentine as an antitubercular agent cannot be recommended for patients taking antiretrovirals at this time due to lack of efficacy data [7, 8]. In all cases, close monitoring and dosage adjustments must accompany all patients being treated concurrently for both conditions.

A special consideration for the co-treatment of these conditions is the development of immune reconstitution inflammatory syndrome [7]. This phenomenon typically presents as a worsening of tuberculosis syndromes after initiation of antiretroviral therapy. However, symptoms tend to be alleviated as treatment continues with only additional symptomatic treatment when applicable. Therefore, both antiretroviral and tuberculosis treatment regimens should be continued while patients are being managed [7].

2.2   Malaria

Malaria is one of the most common infectious diseases worldwide and affects millions of adults and children each year [9]. Malaria typically occurs in areas of sub-Saharan Africa and Asia where HIV rates are also high. Therefore, patients with these comorbidities are at risk from actual and potential drug interactions between antimalarials and antiretrovirals [2]. Although treatment duration with antimalarials is typically short (up to 1 week), this is more than enough time for alteration of the pharmacokinetics and pharmacodynamics of concurrently used agents.

First-line regimens used to treat malaria are artemisinin-based combination therapies (ACTs) [9]. These regimens consist of a primary artemisinin agent (artemisinin, artemether, dihydroartemisinin, artesunate) and a combination agent (lumefantrine, piperaquine, amodiaquine, sulfadoxine- pyrimethamine, mefloquine, or others). Quinine also remains first-line treatment for those patients presenting with severe malaria. The multidrug regimens, along with the pharmacokinetic and pharmacodynamic properties of each individual agent, increase propensity for interactions with antiretrovirals [2].

While pharmacodynamic interactions do exist, there are more data detailing pharmacokinetic interactions with ACTs. A recent systematic review found that ACTs are more vulnerable to the effects of antiretrovirals, rather than vice versa [10]. This finding means antimalarial regimens are likely prone to therapeutic failure or greater toxicity when co-administered with antiretroviral agents. However, the clinical applications of this finding are currently unclear. Specific interaction details are given throughout the remaining chapters of this book.

2.3   Hepatitis B and C

Co-infection with hepatitis B virus (HBV) and/or hepatitis C virus (HCV) increases polypharmacy and potential for drug-drug interactions. HBV and HCV affect up to 20% and 15% of people living with HIV, respectively [2]. A large majority of those coinfected with HCV are patients who inject drugs [11]. Treatment durations for both HBV and HCV are long, and therefore, extra caution must be given when selecting agents in terms of overlapping toxicities and long-term effects. However, many drugs used to treat HIV are also used to treat HBV and therefore interaction potential can be minimized [12].

The recent advances in HCV treatment with respect to direct-acting antiviral agents have resulted in many new agents with potential pharmacokinetic and pharmacodynamic drug-drug interactions with HIV antiretrovirals [13]. Although some data exist to help guide therapeutic decisions, the lack of experience combining these agents precludes firm conclusions to be made regarding regimen safety. Therefore, any patient receiving concurrent treatment for HCV and HIV must be carefully assessed and monitored for both efficacy and safety. Further discussion regarding known interactions with agents used to treat both HBV and HCV is given in subsequent chapters.

2.4 Mental Health Disorders

Patients with HIV are at risk of mental health disorders, including depression, anxiety, dementia, and substance use disorders [2]. These conditions must be taken very seriously and treated appropriately. Coexisting mental health disorders have the ability to affect HIV treatment and adherence rates, and therefore, drug regimens must be carefully selected [14]. Additionally, substance use disorders can also place patients and others at risk due to harmful behaviors. Patient education and counseling are also core components of treatment for these patients.

Mental health and substance use treatment consists of a variety of drug classes that each has side effects and potential pharmacokinetic drug interactions. Due to the difficulty in treating mental health disorders, polypharmacy is often used as a primary therapeutic strategy [15]. Unfortunately, this increases chances of interactions with antiretroviral agents and may lead to compromised efficacy and safety. Aside from pharmacokinetic interactions, overlapping toxicities of these agents, as well as recreational drugs, must be considered when prescribed in conjunction with antiretrovirals [16]. Central nervous system, hepatic, and cardiac toxicities are of particular concern. Further discussion regarding these considerations is presented in subsequent chapters.

2.5 Summary

HIV patients are at increased risk of polypharmacy and associated drug interactions from common comorbidities associated with infection. Many of these are context or regional specific (i.e., malaria, substance use), but others are applicable to all populations. Special attention must be given to patients presenting with comorbidities, especially as HIV therapy transitions to be chronic in nature. Potential for pharmacokinetic and pharmacodynamic drug interactions, including overlapping toxicities, must be carefully assessed, monitored, and followed up over time. This is especially important in regions with increasing drug access and capability to treat common comorbidities associated with HIV infection.

References

1. Marzolini C, Elzi L, Gibbons S, Weber R, Fux C, Furrer H et al (2010) Prevalence of comedications and effect of potential drug-drug interactions in the Swisss HIV Cohort Study. Antivir Ther 15(3):413–423
2. World Health Organization (WHO). Chapter 8: Clinical guidance across the continuum of care: managing common coinfections and comorbidities. In: Consolidated ARV guidelines. 2013. Available from: http://www.who.int/hiv/pub/guidelines/arv2013/coinfection/en/. Accessed 18 June 2016

3. Goulet JL, Fultz SL, Rimland D, Butt A, Gibert C, Rodriguez-Barradas M et al (2007) Do patterns of comorbidity vary by HIV status, age, and HIV severity? Clin Infect Dis 45(12): 1593–1601
4. Nunn P, Williams B, Floyd K, Dye C, Elzinga G, Raviglione M (2005) Tuberculosis control in the era of HIV. Nat Rev Immunol 5(10):819–826
5. World Health Organization (WHO) (2010) Treatment of tuberculosis guidelines, 4th ed. Available from: http://www.who.int/tb/publications/2010/9789241547833/en/. Accessed 18 June 2016
6. Horne DJ, Spitters C, Narita M (2011) Experience with rifabutin replacing rifampin in the treatemnt of tuberculosis. Int J Tuberc Lung Dis 15(11):1485–1489
7. Panel on Antiretroviral Guidelines for Adults and Adolescents. Guidelines for the use of antiretroviral agents in HIV-1 infected adults and adolescents. Department of Health and Human Services. 2016. Available at http://www.aidsinfo.nih.gov/ContentFiles/AdultandAdolescentGL. pdf. Accessed 15 June 2016
8. Centers for Disease Control and Prevention (CDC). Recommendations for the use of an isoniazid-rifapentine regimen with direct observation to treat latent *Mycobacterium tuberculosis* infection. MMWR. Morbidity and mortality weekly reports 2011;60:1650–1653. Available from: http://www.cdc.gov/mmwr/preview/mmwrhtml/mm6048a3.htm. Accessed 19 June 2016
9. World Health Organization (WHO) (2015) Guidelines for the treatment of malaria, 3rd ed. Available from: http://www.who.int/malaria/publications/atoz/9789241549127/en/. Accessed 18 June 2016
10. Kiang TK, Wilby KJ, Ensom MH (2014) Clinical pharmacokinetic drug interactions associated with artemisinin derivatives and HIV-antivirals. Clin Pharmacokinet 53(2):141–153
11. Alter MJ (2006) Epidemiology of viral hepatitis and HIV co-infection. J Hepatol 44(1Suppl):S6–S9
12. Soriano V, Puoti M, Peters M, Benhamou Y, Sulkowski M, Zoulim F et al (2008) Care of HIV patients with chronic hepatitis B: updated recommendations from the HIV-Hepatitis B Virus International Panel. AIDS 22(12):1399–1410
13. El-Sherif O, Back D (2015) Drug interactions of hepatitis C direct-acting antivirals in the HIV-infected person. Curr HIV/AIDS Rep 12(3):336–343
14. Catz SL, Kelly JA, Bogart LM, Benotsch EG, McAuliffe TL (2000) Patterns, correlates, and barriers to medication adherence among persons prescribed new treatments for HIV disease. Health Psychol 19(2):124–133
15. Mojtabai R, Olfson M (2010) National trends in psychotropic medication polypharmacy in office-based psychiatry. Arch Gen Psychiatry 67(1):26–36
16. Gruber VA, McCance-Katz EF (2010) Methadone, buprenorphine, and street drug interactions with antiretroviral medications. Curr HIV/AIDS Rep 7(3):152–160
17. DeSilva KE, Le Flore DB, Marston BJ, Rimland D (2001) Serotonin syndrome in HIV-infected individuals receiving antiretroviral therapy and fluoxetine. AIDS 15(10):1281–1285

Chapter 3
Pharmacology and Pharmacokinetic Properties of Available Antiretrovirals

Kyle John Wilby, Tony K.L. Kiang, and Mary H.H. Ensom

Currently recommended antiretrovirals consist of a variety of agents from different drug classes. Differences in mechanism of action result in unique combinations that allow for additive interactions and synergy, leading to increased therapeutic success. However, overlapping toxicities place patients at risk of increased adverse effects such as hepatotoxicity and endocrine abnormalities. A summary of the pharmacological and pharmacokinetic considerations is given in Table 3.1 for currently available nucleoside reverse transcriptase inhibitors, nonnucleoside reverse transcriptase inhibitors, protease inhibitors, entry inhibitors, fusion inhibitors, integrase inhibitors, and pharmacokinetic enhancers.

K.J. Wilby
College of Pharmacy, Qatar University, Doha, Qatar
e-mail: kjw@qu.edu.qa

T.K.L. Kiang • M.H.H. Ensom (✉)
Faculty of Pharmaceutical Sciences, The University of British Columbia,
Vancouver, BC, Canada
e-mail: tkiang@gmail.com; mary.ensom@ubc.ca

© Springer Science+Business Media Singapore 2016   15
T.K.L. Kiang et al. (eds.), *Pharmacokinetic and Pharmacodynamic Drug Interactions Associated with Antiretroviral Drugs*,
DOI 10.1007/978-981-10-2113-8_3

Table 3.1 Pharmacology and pharmacokinetic properties of antiretrovirals

Class	Drug and reference	Mechanism of action	Clinical pharmacology	Special considerations
Nucleoside reverse transcriptase inhibitors	Abacavir (ABC) [1, 2]	Guanosine analogue which interferes with HIV viral RNA-dependent DNA polymerase resulting in inhibition of viral replication	*Absorption:* rapid and extensive *Distribution:* Vd 0.86 L/kg, 50 % protein bound *Metabolism:* Hepatic via alcohol dehydrogenase and glucuronosyltransferase *Elimination:* Half-life 1.5 h, excreted primarily in urine as metabolites	Hypersensitivity more common in patients positive for *HLA-B*5701* allele Contraindicated in moderate-to-severe hepatic impairment
	Didanosine (ddI) [1, 2]	Purine (adenosine) nucleoside analogue converted to mono- di- and tri-phosphates of dideoxyadenosine that inhibit HIV reverse transcriptase and block viral DNA synthesis	*Absorption:* degradation by acidic pH, ≤50 % reduction in peak plasma concentration in presence of food *Distribution:* Vd 1.08 L/kg, <5 % protein bound *Metabolism:* Not evaluated in humans *Elimination:* Elimination half-life 1.5 h, excreted in urine (55 % as unchanged drug)	Use limited by adverse effects (peripheral neuropathy, diarrhea, other gastrointestinal complaints) Increased risk of pancreatitis (dose-related)
	Emtricitabine (FTC) [1, 2]	Cytosine analogue phosphorylated intracellularly to emtricitabine 5′-triphosphate that interferes with HIV viral RNA dependant DNA polymerase	*Absorption:* rapid, extensive *Distribution:* <4 % protein bound *Metabolism:* limited metabolism via oxidation and conjugation *Elimination:* elimination half-life = 10 h, 86 % excreted unchanged in urine	Potential for exacerbation of hepatitis B after discontinuation of FTC
	Lamivudine (3TC) [1, 2]	Cytosine analogue that is triphosphorylated and inhibits HIV reverse transcriptase via viral DNA chain termination and also inhibits RNA- and DNA-dependent DNA polymerase	*Absorption:* rapid *Distribution:* Vd 1.3 L/kg, <36 % protein bound *Metabolism:* 4.2 % to trans-sulfoxide metabolite *Elimination:* elimination half-life 5–7 h, primarily excreted in urine as unchanged drug	Also indicated for treatment of hepatitis B

Drug	Mechanism	Pharmacokinetics	Major side effects
Stavudine (d4T) [1, 2]	Thymidine analogue that interferes with HIV viral DNA dependent DNA polymerase	*Absorption:* *Distribution:* Vd 46 L *Metabolism:* intracellular phosphorylation to active metabolite *Elimination:* elimination half-life 1.2–1.6 h, 42 % excreted in urine as unchanged drug	Major side effects of peripheral neuropathy and gastrointestinal complaints Increased pancreatitis risk when used with didanosine
Tenofovir (TDF) [1, 2]	Adenosine 5′-monophosphate analogue that interferes with HIV viral RNA dependent DNA polymerase and inhibits viral replication	*Absorption:* *Distribution:* 1.2–1.3 L/kg, $\leq 7\%$ bound to plasma proteins *Metabolism:* tenofovir disoproxil fumarate converted intracellularly to tenofovir through hydrolysis and then phosphorylated to active tenofovir diphosphate *Elimination:* elimination half-life 17 h, 70–80 % excreted in urine primarily as unchanged tenofovir	Also indicated for hepatitis B and acute exacerbation may occur upon discontinuation Caution in renal dysfunction
Zidovudine (AZT) [1, 2]	Thymidine analogue that interferes with HIV viral RNA-dependent DNA polymerase, inhibiting viral replication	*Absorption:* *Distribution:* Vd 1–2.2 L/kg, significant penetration into CSF, crosses placenta, 25–38 % protein bound *Metabolism:* hepatically metabolized via glucuronidation to inactive metabolites *Elimination:* elimination half-life 0.5–3 h, 72–74 % excreted in urine as metabolites and 14–18 % as unchanged drug	Major hematologic toxicity including granulocytopenia, severe anemia or pancytopenia Prolonged use associated with myopathy and myositis

(continued)

Table 3.1 (continued)

Class	Drug and reference	Mechanism of action	Clinical pharmacology	Special considerations
Non-nucleoside reverse transcriptase inhibitors	Delavirdine (DLV) [1, 3]	Binds directly to HIV reverse transcriptase and blocks RNA-dependent and DNA-dependent DNA polymerase activity	*Absorption*: rapid *Distribution*: approximately 98 % bound to serum albumin *Metabolism*: hepatic via CYP314 and 2D6 *Elimination*: elimination half-life 5.8 h, 51 % excreted in urine (<5 % as unchanged drug) and 44 % excreted in feces	Demonstrates non-linear kinetics May induce own metabolism
	Efavirenz (EFV) [1, 4]	Binds to HIV reverse transcriptase and blocks RNA-dependent and DNA-dependent DNA polymerase activities	*Absorption*: increased by fatty meals *Distribution*: >99 % protein bound (albumin) *Metabolism*: hepatic metabolism via CYP3A4 and 2B6 to inactive hydroxylated metabolites *Elimination*: elimination half-life 40–55 h with multiple doses, excreted in feces as unchanged drug (16–61 %) and urine as metabolites (14–34 %)	Does not require intracellular phosphorylation May induce own metabolism CNS and dermatologic adverse reactions common
	Etravirine (ETV) [1, 5]	Binds to reverse transcriptase and blocks RNA-dependent and DNA-dependent DNA polymerase activities including viral replication	*Absorption*: increased 50% with food *Distribution*: 99.9 % protein bound to albumin and alpha$_1$-acid glycoprotein *Metabolism*: hepatic via CYP3A4, 2C9, and 2C19 to metabolites with approximately 10% of parent drug activity *Elimination*: elimination half-life 41 h, excreted in feces (94 %, up to 86 % as unchanged drug) and urine (1 %)	Does not require intracellular phosphorylation Dermatological and endocrine adverse reactions High potential for drug interactions

	Nevirapine (NVP) [1, 4]	Binds to reverse transcriptase and blocks RNA-dependent and DNA-dependent DNA polymerase activities including viral replication	*Absorption:* >90 % *Distribution:* 1.2–1.4 L/kg, 60 % protein bound *Metabolism:* hepatic via CYP3A4 to inactive compounds, may undergo enterohepatic recycling *Elimination:* elimination half-life 25–30 h (with chronic dosing after autoinduction), excreted in urine (81 %, primarily as metabolites) and feces (10 %)	Severe hepatotoxic reactions may occur Severe skin reactions (Stevens-Johnson syndrome, toxic epidermal necrolysis) may occur and must be monitored within first 18 weeks of therapy
	Rilpivirine (RPV) [1]	Binds to reverse transcriptase and blocks RNA-dependent and DNA-dependent DNA polymerase activities including viral replication	*Absorption:* increases 40 % with a normal to high calorie meal *Distribution:* 99.7 % protein bound primarily to albumin *Metabolism:* hepatic via CYP3A4 *Elimination:* elimination half-life approximately 50 h, excreted in feces (85 %, 25 % as unchanged drug) and urine (6 %, <1 % unchanged drug)	Limited information available for renal and hepatic failure Contraindicated with coadministration with anticonvulsants (induces CYP3A4) Primarily neurological, gastrointestinal, and endocrine adverse reactions
Protease inhibitors	Atazanavir (ATV) [1, 6, 7]	Inhibits HIV-1 protease which prevents cleavage of gag-pol polyprotein resulting in production of immature non-infectious virus	*Absorption:* rapid, enhanced with food *Distribution:* 86 % protein bound *Metabolism:* hepatic via multiple pathways including CYP3A4 *Elimination:* elimination half-life 7–8 h (unboosted), 9–18 h (boosted)	Caution in patients with pre-existing cardiac conduction abnormalities

(continued)

Table 3.1 (continued)

Class	Drug and reference	Mechanism of action	Clinical pharmacology	Special considerations
	Darunavir (DRV) [1, 7]	Inhibits HIV-1 protease which prevents cleavage of gag-pol polyprotein resulting in production of immature non-infectious virus	*Absorption:* increased 30 % with food *Distribution:* 95 % protein bound *Metabolism:* hepatic via CYP3A4 *Elimination:* elimination half-life 15 h (boosted), 80 % excreted in feces (41 % as unchanged drug), 14 % excreted in urine (8 % as unchanged drug)	Co-administration with ritonavir required May cause fat redistribution and other lipid abnormalities
	Fosamprenavir (FPV) [1, 7]	Inhibits HIV-1 protease which prevents cleavage of gag-pol polyprotein resulting in production of immature non-infectious virus	*Absorption:* 63 % *Distribution:* >90 % bound to apha$_1$-acid glycoprotein *Metabolism:* converted to amprenavir by cellular phosphates, amprenavir hepatically metabolized by CYP3A4 (primarily) *Elimination:* amprenavir elimination half-life 7.7 h, excreted in feces (75 % as metabolites), and urine (14 % as metabolites)	Rapidly converted to amprenavir (active moiety) by cellular phosphates
	Indinavir (IDV) [1, 7]	Inhibits HIV-1 protease which prevents cleavage of polyproteins resulting in production of immature non-infectious virus	*Absorption:* high fat diet decreases AUC and Cmax (77 % and 84 %, respectively) *Distribution:* 60 % protein bound *Metabolism:* hepatic via CYP3A4 *Elimination:* elimination half-life 1.8 h, 83 % excreted in feces (19 % unchanged) and 19 % excreted in urine (9 % as unchanged)	May cause nephrolithiasis/urolithiasis Gastrointestinal, hepatic, and renal adverse effects most common

Nelfinavir (NFV) [1, 7]	Inhibits HIV-1 protease which prevents cleavage of gag-pol polyprotein resulting in production of immature non-infectious virus	*Absorption:* increased 2–5 fold with food *Distribution:* Vd 2–7 L/kg *Metabolism:* hepatic via CYP2C19 and 3A4 *Elimination:* elimination half-life 3.5–5 h, 98–99 % excreted in feces (78 % as metabolites, 22 % as unchanged drug)	Active major metabolite
Ritonavir (RTV) [1, 7]	Inhibits HIV-1 protease which prevents cleavage of gag-pol polyprotein resulting in production of immature non-infectious virus	*Absorption:* increases with food *Distribution:* Vd 0.16–0.66 L/kg, 98–99 % protein bound *Metabolism:* hepatic via CYP3A4 and 2D6 *Elimination:* elimination half-life 3–5 h, excreted 11 % in urine (4 % unchanged), 86 % in feces (34 % unchanged)	Used to boost other protease inhibitor concentrations through enzyme inhibition Endocrine, gastrointestinal, hepatic, and neuromuscular/skeletal adverse effects most common
Saquinavir (SQV) [1, 7]	Inhibits HIV protease by preventing cleavage of viral polyprotein precursors needed to generate functional viral proteins needed for maturation of virus	*Absorption:* poor but increased with high fat meal *Distribution:* Vd 700 L, 98 % protein bound *Metabolism:* extensively metabolized hepatically by CYP3A4 *Elimination:* 81–88 % in feces, 1–3 % in urine	Caution in patients with hepatic dysfunction

(continued)

Table 3.1 (continued)

Class	Drug and reference	Mechanism of action	Clinical pharmacology	Special considerations
	Tipranavir (TPV) [1, 7]	Non-peptide inhibitor of HIV-1 protease by binding to activity site and inhibits enzyme activity, resulting in formation of immature and non-infectious viral particles	*Absorption:* incomplete but undetermined. *Distribution:* Vd 7.7–10 L, >99 % protein bound. *Metabolism:* hepatic via CYP3A4 (minimal when boosted with RTV). *Elimination:* elimination half-life 6 h, 82 % excreted in feces, 4 % excreted in urine (primarily unchanged when boosted with RTV)	When boosted with ritonavir, may cause hepatic dysfunction. Associated with rare reports of intracranial hemorrhage
	Lopinavir (LPV) [1, 7]	Inhibits HIV protease and renders enzyme incapable of processing polyprotein precursor, which leads to production of immature and non-infectious HIV particles	*Absorption:* *Distribution:* 98–99 % protein bound. *Metabolism:* hepatic via CYP3A4. *Elimination:* elimination half-life 5–6 h, 83 % excreted in feces (20 % unchanged) and 10 % excreted in urine (<3 % unchanged)	Always administered with ritonavir. Caution endocrine and hepatic adverse effects
Fusion inhibitors	Enfuvirtide (T-20) [1]	Binds first heptad-repeat (HR1) in gp41 subunit of viral envelope glycoprotein and inhibits fusion of HIV virus with CD4 cells by blocking conformational change in gp41 required for membrane fusion and entry	*Absorption:* *Distribution:* Vd 5.5 L. *Metabolism:* metabolized by proteolytic hydrolysis. *Excretion:* elimination half-life 3.8 h	Subcutaneous injection. Associated with increases in pneumonia

Entry inhibitors	Maraviroc (MVC) [1, 8]	Selectively and reversibly binds to chemokine CCR5 located on CD4 cells and prevents interaction between CCR5 co-receptor and gp120 subunit of viral envelope glycoprotein inhibiting conformational change required for HIV fusion with CD4 cell and subsequent cell entry	Absorption: Distribution: Vd 194 L, 76 % protein bound Metabolism: hepatic via CYP3A to inactive metabolites Elimination: elimination half-life 14–18 h, 20 % excreted in urine (8 % as unchanged) and 76 % excreted in feces (25 % as unchanged drug)	Possible drug induced hepatotoxicity with allergic features Fever and respiratory tract infections most common adverse effects
Integrase inhibitors	Dolutegravir (DTG) [1, 9]	Binds to integrase active site and inhibits strand transfer of HIV DNA integration necessary for HIV replication	Absorption: food increases extent and slows rate of absorption (up to 66 % with high fat meals) Distribution: Vd/F = 17.4 L, >98 % protein bound Metabolism: primarily metabolized by UGT1A1 and less so by CYP3A Elimination: elimination half-life of 14 h, excreted in feces (53 % as unchanged), and urine (31 % as metabolites, <1 % unchanged)	Recommended to administer without regard to meals Endocrine and hepatic adverse events most common
	Elvitegravir (EVG) [1, 10]	Inhibits catalytic activity of integrase, preventing integration of proviral gene into human DNA	Absorption: AUC increases with food Distribution: 99 % protein bound Metabolism: hepatic via CYP3A and glucuronidated by UGT1A1/3 Elimination: elimination half-life of 9 h, excreted in feces (95 %) and urine (7 %)	Neurological and gastrointestinal adverse effects most common Limited information in hepatic impairment

(continued)

Table 3.1 (continued)

Class	Drug and reference	Mechanism of action	Clinical pharmacology	Special considerations
	Raltegravir (RAL) [1]	Inhibits catalytic activity of integrase, preventing integration of proviral gene into human DNA	*Absorption:* high fat meal increases AUC 19 % *Distribution:* 83 % protein bound *Metabolism:* hepatic glucuronidation by UGT1A1 *Elimination:* elimination half-life 9 h, excreted in feces (51 %) and urine (32 %)	Endocrine and metabolic adverse effects most common
Pharmacokinetic enhancers	Cobicistat (COBI or C) [1]	Mechanism-based inhibitor of CYP3A in order to increase systemic exposure of paired CYP3A substrates such as atazanavir and darunavir	*Absorption:* – *Distribution:* 97–98 % protein bound *Metabolism:* primarily by CYP3A enzymes and CYP2D6 without glucuronidation *Elimination:* elimination half-life of 3–4 h	High potential for drug interactions through CYP3A inhibition May cause renal toxicity when co-administered with tenofovir

AUC area-under-the curve, *Cmax* maximum concentration, *CYP* cytochrome P450, *HIV* human immunodeficiency virus, *UGT* UDP-glucuronosyltransferase, *Vd* volume of distribution

References

1. Lexi-comp (2015) Drug information handbook, 24th edn. Lexi-comp, Inc, Hudson
2. Piliero PJ (2004) Pharmacokinetic properties of nucleoside/nucleotide reverse transcriptase inhibitors. J Acquir Immune Defic Syndr 37(Suppl 1):S2–S12
3. Tran JQ, Gerber JG, Kerr BM (2001) Delavirdine: clinical pharmacokinetics and drug interactions. Clin Pharmacokinet 40(3):207–226
4. Smith PF, DiCenzo R, Morse GD (2001) Clinical pharmacokinetics of non-nucleoside reverse transcriptase inhibitors. Clin Pharmacokinet 40(12):893–905
5. Scholler-Gyure M, Kakuda TN, Raoof A, De Smedt G, Hoetelmans RMW (2009) Clinical pharmacokinetics and pharmacodynamics of etravirine. Clin Pharmacokinet 48(9):561–574
6. Le Tiec C, Barrail A, Goujard C, Taburet A (2005) Clinical pharmacokinetics and summary of efficacy and tolerability of atazanavir. Clin Pharmacokinet 44(10):1035–1050
7. Flexner C (1998) HIV-protease inhibitors. N Eng J Med 338(18):1281–1293
8. Abel S, Back DJ, Vourvahis M (2009) Maraviroc: pharmacokinetics and drug interactions. Antivir Ther 14(5):607–618
9. Cottrell ML, Hadzic T, Kashuba AD (2013) Clinical pharmacokinetic, pharmacodynamic and drug-interaction profile of the integrase inhibitor dolutegravir. Clin Pharmacokinet 52(11):981–994
10. Ramanathan S, Mathias AA, German P, Kearney BP (2011) Clinical pharmacokinetic and pharmacodynamic profile of the HIV integrase inhibitor elvitegravir. Clin Pharmacokinet 50(4):229–244

Chapter 4
In Vitro Reaction Phenotyping and Drug Interaction Data

Tony K.L. Kiang, Kyle John Wilby, and Mary H.H. Ensom

This chapter summarizes the in vitro reaction phenotyping and drug interaction data for each antiretroviral agent. Investigations on the relative contributions of specific metabolizing enzymes and molecular enzyme inhibition/induction reactions will be presented for the following agents, based on drug class:

Nonnucleoside reverse transcriptase inhibitors (NNRTIs): delavirdine, efavirenz, etravirine, nevirapine, and rilpivirine

Nucleoside reverse-transcriptase inhibitors (NRTIs): abacavir, didanosine, emtric-itabine, lamivudine, stavudine, tenofovir, and zidovudine

Protease inhibitors (PIs): atazanavir, darunavir, fosamprenavir, indinavir, nelfinavir, ritonavir, saquinavir, tipranavir, and lopinavir

Fusion inhibitors: enfuvirtide

Entry inhibitors: maraviroc

Integrase inhibitors: dolutegravir, elvitegravir, raltegravir

---

T.K.L. Kiang • M.H.H. Ensom (✉)
Faculty of Pharmaceutical Sciences, The University of British Columbia,
Vancouver, BC, Canada
e-mail: tkiang@gmail.com; mary.ensom@ubc.ca

K.J. Wilby
College of Pharmacy, Qatar University, Doha, Qatar
e-mail: kjw@qu.edu.qa

© Springer Science+Business Media Singapore 2016   27
T.K.L. Kiang et al. (eds.), *Pharmacokinetic and Pharmacodynamic Drug Interactions Associated with Antiretroviral Drugs*,
DOI 10.1007/978-981-10-2113-8_4

4.1 Nonnucleoside Reverse Transcriptase Inhibitors

4.1.1 Delavirdine

In humans, delavirdine is primarily metabolized in the liver by cytochrome P450 (CYP) 3A4 and to a minor extent by CYP2D6 in humans. This is based on the study by Voorman et al. [1] which showed significant correlations between delavirdine desalkylation and testosterone 6-beta-hydroxylation (a marker reaction for CYP3A) in human liver microsomes. In support of the correlational study, only CYP3A4 and CYP2D6 were able to catalyze the oxidation of delavirdine in a panel of 11 cDNA-expressed supersomes. These observations were supported by chemical inhibition experiments using ketoconazole and troleandomycin (selective CYP3A4 inhibitors), which showed extensive attenuation of delavirdine desalkylation in human liver microsomes, indicating a primary role for CYP3A4. On the other hand, quinidine (selective CYP2D6 inhibitor) had little effects on delavirdine desalkylation in human liver microsomes, suggesting a relatively minor contribution to this specific reaction.

In addition to being a substrate for CYP3A4, delavirdine is known to inhibit the enzyme in a mechanistic manner [2] as demonstrated in human liver microsomes using triazolam as the CYP3A4 marker substrate (with inhibitory constant (Ki) of ~21.6 μM). In a separate study [3], delavirdine also demonstrated inhibition against CYP2C9 (using diclofenac as substrate marker, Ki ~2.6 μM, in human liver microsomes), CYP2C19 (using (S)-mephenytoin as substrate marker, Ki ~24 μM, in cDNA-expressed CYP2C19 supersomes), and CYP2D6 (using dextromethorphan as substrate marker, Ki ~13 μM, in cDNA-expressed CYP2D6 supersomes). These findings suggest that delavirdine can potentially reduce the metabolism of CYP3A4, CYP2C9, CYP2C19, and CYP2D6 substrates. The exact mechanisms of inhibition, other than that documented for CYP3A4, remain to be investigated.

4.1.2 Efavirenz

In vitro reaction phenotyping studies indicate that CYP2B6 and UDP-glucuronosyltransferase (UGT) 2B7 are the primary enzymes responsible for the oxidation of efavirenz in humans. Using a panel of cDNA-expressed human supersomes, Ward et al. [4] found that CYP2B6 catalyzed the formation of efavirenz metabolites with the highest activities, which is supported by significant inhibition of efavirenz oxidation by triethylenethiophosphoramide (selective inhibitor of CYP2B6) in human liver microsomes. Using a panel of expressed UGT enzymes, only UGT2B7 demonstrated catalytic activity toward the formation of efavirenz-N-glucuronide [5], which corresponds with the observed inhibition of efavirenz glucuronidation by 3'-azido-3'deoxythymidine (AZT), a probe substrate for UGT2B7.

Efavirenz is an inducer of CYP3A4, as demonstrated in primary human hepato-cytes using testosterone 6-beta hydroxylation as the marker reaction [6]. The extent of CYP3A4 induction by efavirenz (~3-fold) is comparable to that of the prototypi-cal inducer, rifampin (~4-fold), indicating a likely to be clinically significant effect. In addition to inducing CYP3A4 activity, in vitro experiments also indicate that efavirenz can activate the enzyme, as demonstrated by increased rates of midazolam 1′-hydroxlation in human liver microsomes [7]. On the other hand, efavirenz is known to inhibit CYP and UGT enzymes. In human liver microsomes, efavirenz was shown to be a competitive inhibitor of CYP2B6 (Ki ~1.7 μM), CYP2C8 (Ki ~4.8 μM), CYP2C9 (Ki ~19.5 μM), and CYP2C19 (Ki ~21.3 μM). With respect to UGT enzymes, efavirenz has been shown to potently inhibit the glucuronidation of trifluoperazine (a marker substrate for UGT1A4, Ki ~2 μM), propofol (a marker substrate for UGT1A9, Ki ~9 μM) [8], and AZT (a marker substrate for UBT2B7, Ki ~17 μM) [5]. Based on these findings, the plasma exposure of drug substrates metabolized by these enzyme systems may be modulated when co-administered with efavirenz.

4.1.3   Etravirine

In human liver microsomes, etravirine is primarily metabolized by CYP2C19 and CYP3A4/5 [9]. In a panel of cDNA-expressed CYP450 supersomes, only CYP3A4/5 and CYP2C19 showed significant catalytic activities toward the oxidation of etra-virine. The primary roles of CYP2C19 and CYP3A4 in etravirine metabolism are supported by chemical inhibition experiments demonstrating significant reductions in metabolite formation when etravirine is co-incubated with (+)-N-3-benzylnirvanol and ketoconazole, which are selective inhibitors for CYP2C19 and CYP3A4, respectively, in human liver microsomes. By virtue of etravirine being a substrate of these CYP450 enzymes, it can theoretically act as a competitive inhibitor, although systematic inhibition experiments are still lacking. On the other hand, etravirine has been shown to enhance CYP3A4 mRNA expression in primary human hepatocytes in a time-dependent manner, possibly mediated by the pregnane X receptor [9].

4.1.4   Nevirapine

Nevirapine is extensively metabolized in the liver by CYP3A4 and CYP2B6 enzymes. Four primary metabolites of nevirapine have been identified in vitro (2-, 3-, 8-, and 12-hydroxy nevirapine), and their formations are catalyzed predomi-nately by either CY3A4 or CYP2B6, as demonstrated in a panel of cDNA-expressed CYP450 supersomes [10]. This observation is supported by significant reductions in metabolite formation when nevirapine is co-incubated with enzyme-specific inhibi-tory antibodies or selective chemical inhibitors (i.e., ketoconazole, troleandomycin, erythromycin) toward CYP3A4 and CYP2B6 in human liver microsomes. Despite being a substrate for these enzymes, nevirapine was shown to exhibit little inhibitory activity toward CYP3A4 and CYP2B6 or to other CYP450 enzymes (CYP1A2, CYP2A6, CYP2C9, CYP2C19, CYP2D6, and CYP2E1) using selective probe substrate markers in human liver microsomes [10]. In contrast to other NNRTIs, the induction capability of nevirapine toward CYP enzymes has not been well characterized in human in vitro systems.

4.1.5   *Rilpivirine*

Rilpivirine oxidation is primarily catalyzed by CYP3A4/5 and conjugated by UGT1A1 or UGT1A4 in the formation of various metabolites in the human liver [11]. In a panel of cDNA-expressed CYPs and UGTs, only CYP1A2, CYP2C19, CYP3A4/5, UGT1A1, and UGT1A4 showed significant activities toward the oxidation or conjugation of rilpivirine. Chemical inhibition experiments using a panel of CYP selective inhibitors indicated that ketoconazole (CYP3A4/5 inhibitor) but not furafylline (CYP1A2 inhibitor) co-incubation resulted in the greatest reductions in the formation of rilpivirine oxidative metabolites, confirming a relatively major role of CYP3A4 in the oxidative metabolism of rilpivirine. Because chemical or antibody-mediated inhibitions have not been conducted for UGT enzymes, the relative contributions of UGT1A1 and UGT1A4 to the glucuronidation of rilpivirine remain to be determined in future studies. Rilpivirine has been shown to inhibit CYP3A4, CYP2C19, and CYP2B6 in vitro and induce the expression of CYP3A4 and UGT1A3 mRNAs in LS180 cells [12], suggesting potentials for enzyme-mediated drug-drug interactions. However, further studies are needed to characterize the interaction potential of rilpivirine (i.e., determination of Ki values and the mechanisms of inhibition) in human hepatic models (e.g., primary cultures of human hepatocytes). Otherwise, extensive drug-drug interaction studies have not been reported for rilpivirine.

4.2   Nucleoside Reverse-Transcriptase Inhibitors

4.2.1   *Abacavir*

Abacavir is not metabolized by CYP450 enzymes. In humans, mass balance studies indicate that abacavir is carboxylated and glucuronidated by alcohol dehydrogenase and UGT enzymes, respectively [13]. However, the exact identities of the metabolites and the relative contributions of specific enzymes in these reactions have not been characterized. Little information is available on the drug-interaction potential of abacavir. However, it is unlikely that abacavir would mediate drug-drug interactions via CYP450 enzymes because it is not a substrate of this enzyme system.

4.2.2   Didanosine

Little information on the metabolic fate of didanosine has been published in the literature. One might speculate that it may undergo similar metabolic patterns as purines due to similar chemistry in humans. Likewise, little data on the drug-drug interaction potential of didanosine have been made available.

4.2.3   Emtricitabine, Lamivudine, Stavudine, Tenofovir

Emtricitabine, lamivudine, stavudine, and tenofovir are primarily cleared (unchanged) by renal excretion and undergo very minimal hepatic biotransformation [14]. As such, metabolic enzyme-mediated drug interactions are unlikely to be associated with these agents. Tenofovir has been shown to inhibit the metabolism of marker substrates for CYP2C9 (Ki ~420 µM) and CYP2E1 (Ki ~140 µM) in human liver microsomes [15]. However, these nonpotent inhibitory effects are not likely to be clinically relevant due to the high Ki values (i.e., nonattainable plasma concentrations) reported.

4.2.4   Zidovudine

Zidovudine is primarily conjugated by UGT2B7 in the formation of the inactive glucuronide, as demonstrated using a panel of expressed UGT2B enzymes of which only UGT2B7 showed significant catalytic activity in the formation of zidovudine glucuronide [16]. This experiment, however, does not rule out other UGT subfamilies (such as UGT1A) in the glucuronidation of zidovudine. The role of UGT as the predominant enzyme responsible for zidovudine metabolism was further demonstrated in human liver microsomes where known inhibitors of UGT (e.g., atovaquone, fluconazole, methadone, valproic acid, and efavirenz) were able to reduce the glucuronidation of zidovudine in a concentration-dependent manner [5, 17]. These data suggest that zidovudine may be subject to clinically significant drug-drug interactions mediated by UGT2B7 modulators.

Moreover, zidovudine also undergoes metabolism by CYP450 enzymes in the formation of 3′-azido-3′-deoxythymidine in the human liver [18], but the exact identities of the enzymes involved remain to be identified [19]. Despite the use of human liver microsomes, selective CYP450 chemical inhibitors, and specific CYP450 inhibitory antibodies, no definitive conclusions have yet been drawn about the relative contributions of specific CYP450 enzymes involved in zidovudine metabolism. As such, little information is available on the in vitro drug molecular interaction potential of zidovudine.

4.3 Protease Inhibitors

4.3.1 Atazanavir

Atazanavir is primarily metabolized by CYP3A4 in humans as demonstrated in experiments conducted by the manufacturer in human liver microsomes using keto-conazole and troleandomycin as chemical selective inhibitors for the enzyme [20]. A high correlation between the catalytic activity of CYP3A4 toward atazanavir oxida-tion and that of testosterone hydroxylation (marker reaction for CYP3A4) further confirms the primary role of CYP3A4 in atazanavir metabolism. These data are sup-ported by the observation that chemical inhibitors selective for other CYP450 enzymes did not reduce the oxidation of atazanavir [20]. This metabolic profile indicates that atazanavir is likely subjected to drug interactions mediated by CYP3A4 modulators.

In human liver microsomes, atazanavir was shown to inhibit CYP1A2 (Ki ~12 μM), CYP2C9 (Ki ~13 μM), CYP3A4 (Ki ~2 μM), and UGT1A1 in various mechanisms (e.g., competitive or mechanism-based inhibition) [20]. The reported Ki values in these in vitro experiments suggest that the inhibitory effect of atazanavir is potent and may be considered clinically relevant (especially in the case of CYP3A4 substrates). On the other hand, little inhibitory effects of atazanavir have been shown toward CYP2A6, CYP2C19, CYP2D6, CYP2E1, or CYP4A9, and atazanavir has not been known to mediate drug-drug interactions by enzyme induction.

4.3.2 Darunavir

CYP3A4 is the principal enzyme responsible for the metabolism of darunavir in humans. This was based on the observation reported by the manufacturer that only CYP3A4 catalyzed the hydroxylation of darunavir in a panel of cDNA-expressed CYP450 enzymes and that CYP3A4 selective inhibitors (e.g., ketoconazole, trolean-domycin, ritonavir, clarithromycin) were able to significantly reduce the oxidation of darunavir in human liver microsomes [21]. This metabolic characteristic indicates that darunavir is likely to be subjected to drug-drug interactions mediated by CYP3A4 modulators. In addition to being a substrate of CYP3A4, darunavir also inhibits the enzyme in a potent manner (Ki ~0.4 μM), but shows little inhibitory activity toward CYP1A2, CYP2A6, CYP2B6, CYP2C9, CYP2C19, CYP2D6, and CYP2E1 in human liver microsomes, using enzyme selective probe substrates. Little is reported about the enzyme induction potential of darunavir in the literature.

4.3.3 Fosamprenavir

Fosamprenavir is a pro-drug that is rapidly hydrolyzed in the vasculature in the formation of the active moiety, amprenavir, that is, primarily metabolized by CYP3A4 in humans. This was demonstrated in vitro in human liver microsomes

where relatively selective inhibitors of CYP3A4 (ketoconazole, terfenadine, aste-
mizole) were able to significantly inhibit the metabolism of amprenavir [22] and
that only cDNA-expressed CYP3A4 acted as a catalyst, amongst a panel of
enzymes, for amprenavir oxidation. Because it is a substrate of CYP3A4, amprenavir is subject to drug-drug interactions mediated by this enzyme. For example,
various protease inhibitors (e.g., ritonavir, indinavir, nelfinavir, saquinavir) were
shown to inhibit the CYP3A4-catalyzed amprenavir oxidation in human liver
microsomes [22]. Likewise, amprenavir is itself a relatively potent inhibitor of
CYP3A4, as demonstrated by reduced testosterone hydroxylation (Ki ~0.5 μM), a
probe reaction for CYP3A4, in human liver microsomes co-incubated with amprenavir. The mechanism of inhibition has been suggested to be mechanism based or
time-dependent [23].

4.3.4   Indinavir

CYP3A4 is the primary enzyme responsible for the inactivation of indinavir in
humans. The role of CYP3A4 for indinavir oxidation was confirmed by comple-
mentary approaches including a panel of cDNA-expressed CYP450 supersomes
(where CYP3A4 showed highest catalytic activity), selective chemical inhibition
experiments (where ketoconazole and troleandomycin, but not other probe selective
inhibitors, at concentrations selective toward CYP3A4, significantly decreased indinavir oxidation in human liver microsomes), and immune-inhibition (where a
CYP3A4-selective antirat polyclonal antibody that was cross reactive toward human
enzymes significantly reduced the metabolism of indinavir in human liver microsomes) [24]. Indinavir was able to inhibit (Ki ~0.5 μM) testosterone 6-beta-
hydroxylation (marker reaction for CYP3A4), but did not have significant effects on
phenacetin O-deethylation (CYP1A2 marker), tolbutamide hydroxylation (CYP2C9
marker), or chlorzoxazone hydroxylation (CYP2E1 marker) in human liver microsomes [25]. Further supporting the potent inhibitory activity against CYP3A4 substrates, indinavir was shown to competitively inhibit methadone N-demethylation
(Ki ~3 μM), buprenorphine N-dealkylation (Ki ~0.8 μM), and zidovudine oxidation, all substrates for CYP3A4 in human liver microsomes [26, 27]. Mechanism-
based inhibition of CYP3A4 by indinavir has been suggested [28], and little
information on enzyme induction properties of indinavir has been reported.

4.3.5   Nelfinavir

Nelfinavir is metabolized primarily by CYP2C19 in humans in the formation of the
pharmacologically active nelfinavir hydroxyl-t-butylamide. Using a panel of cDNA-
expressed CYP450 enzymes (including CYP2C9, CYP2C8, CYP2C19, and
CYP3A4), only CYP2C19 showed catalytic activity toward the oxidation of nelfinavir [29]. These observations are supported by significant reductions in metabolite

formation when nelfinavir is co-incubated with monoclonal CYP2C19 inhibitory antibody (enzyme specific) or omeprazole (CYP2C19 selective inhibitor) in human liver microsomes, supporting the predominant role of this specific enzyme. With respect to interaction potential, nelfinavir competitively inhibited testosterone 6-beta-hydroxylation, a marker of reaction for CYP3A4 (Ki ~4.8 µM), but had little effects toward CYP2D6, CYP2C19, CYP2C9, CYP2C8, or CYP2E1 marker substrates in human liver microsomes at therapeutically relevant incubation concentrations [30]. The mechanism of CYP3A4 inhibition appeared to be both time- and concentration-dependent and may be potentially clinically relevant given the potency of the inhibition.

4.3.6   Ritonavir

Ritonavir is primarily metabolized by CYP3A4 and CYP2D6 in humans in the formation of various oxidative metabolites. Using cDNA-expressed CYP450 supersomes, only CYP3A and CYP2D6 were able to catalyze the metabolism of ritonavir in vitro [31]. Because the selective chemical inhibitors toward CYP3A4 were not able to completely attenuate the oxidative metabolism of ritonavir in human liver microsomes, some contribution by CYP2D6 in ritonavir metabolism is suggested. Ritonavir itself is a potent inhibitor of CYP1A2, CYP3A4, CYP2D6, and CYP2C9 as evident by its ability to significantly attenuate the oxidation of prototypical substrates for these enzymes [31]. The inhibitory effect of ritonavir toward CYP3A4 is potent, as evident by a Ki of ~0.02 µM, measured by the attenuation of 6-beta-hydroxylation in human liver microsomes [25]. This suggests that ritonavir is likely to mediate clinically relevant drug interactions via CYP3A4 inhibition. On the other hand, ritonavir has also been shown to induce the marker substrate activities and mRNA expressions of various CYP450 enzymes (i.e., CYP1A2, CYP2B6, CYP2C9) and transporters (i.e., organic anion transporter 1B1 and multidrug resistance protein) in human hepatocytes [32]. The complex drug inhibition/induction characteristics of ritonavir likely translate to mixed effects.

4.3.7   Saquinavir

Saquinavir is primarily metabolized by CYP3A4 in humans. This was demonstrated in human liver microsomes where ketoconazole, a selective CYP3A4 chemical inhibitor, was able to decrease the oxidation of saquinavir, whereas selective chemical inhibitors toward other CYP450 enzymes had little effects [33]. Likewise, significant correlations in human liver microsomes between the catalytic activity toward saquinavir and the amount of CYP3A4 (quantified by immunochemistry) or testosterone 6-beta-hydroxylation activity (marker reaction for CYP3A4) were observed. Moreover, protease inhibitors known to inhibit CYP3A4 (ritonavir, indinavir, and nelfinavir) were also capable of reducing the metabolism of saquinavir in human liver microsomes. Taken together, these data support the predominant role of CYP3A4 in saquinavir oxidation in humans.

Saquinavir itself is a potent inhibitor of CYP3A4. In human liver microsomes, saquinavir significantly reduced the formation of 6-beta-hydroxytestosterone (Ki ~0.7 μM) [34], a marker substrate for the enzyme. In the same experimental system, however, ritonavir was relatively more potent (Ki ~0.03 μM) than saquinavir in CYP3A4 inhibition. Moreover, saquinavir was capable of reducing the hydroxylation of tolbutamide (a marker substrate for CYP2C9) in human liver microsomes, but only at concentrations likely not attainable under normal physiological conditions [25]. Similar to ritonavir, saquinavir has been shown to induce the marker substrate activities and mRNA expressions of various CYP450 enzymes and transporters in human hepatocytes [32], resulting in complex drug inhibition and induction profiles when saquinavir is used concurrently with agents metabolized by these enzymes.

4.3.8   Tipranavir

CYP3A4 is the primary enzyme responsible for the metabolism of tipranavir as demonstrated in human liver microsomes using selective chemical inhibitors toward the enzyme (i.e., ketoconazole at 1 μM) and correlational analysis conducted by the manufacturer [35]. Because cDNA-expressed CYP2D6 did not exhibit any catalytic activity toward tipranavir metabolism, it is unlikely this enzyme provides any relative contributions to tipranavir metabolism in humans. Tipranavir inhibits CYP450 enzymes to various degrees of potency, as evident by its effects toward the oxidation of phenacetin (marker for CYP1A2, Ki ~24 μM), diclofenac (CYP2C9, Ki ~0.2 μM), (S)-mephenytoin (CYP2C19, Ki ~5.3 μM), bufuralol (CYP2D6, Ki ~6.7 μM), and testosterone and midazolam (CYP3A4, Ki ~0.9–1.3 μM). The potent inhibitory effects of tipranavir toward CYP2C9 and CYP3A4 suggest potential clinically significant drug-drug interactions when co-administered with substrates for these enzymes. In human hepatocytes, tipranavir was shown to be an inducer of CYP3A4, although its ability to induce other CYP450s or other enzyme systems (e.g., UGT) has not been well characterized. Because it has been demonstrated to be a substrate of p-glycoprotein in vitro (Caco-2 cell permeability assay), transporter-mediated drug-drug interactions should also be considered for tipranavir.

4.3.9   Lopinavir

In vitro studies with human liver microsomes and chemical inhibition experiments indicate that CYP3A4 is the primary enzyme responsible for lopinavir metabolism in humans [35]. Because it is administered only in combination with ritonavir, the drug-interaction potential of the drug pair (rather than lopinavir alone) is usually considered. In vitro experiments conducted by the manufacturer using selective markers for CYP450 in human liver microsomes indicated that the lopinavir/ritonavir combination exhibits similar inhibitory effects toward CYP450 enzymes (i.e., potent inhibition of CYP3A4 with inhibitory effects toward other enzymes) compared to ritonavir administered alone (see above for ritonavir). The mechanism of CYP3A4 inhibition by lopinavir appeared to be mechanism-based and less potent than ritonavir [36]. Ritonavir has been shown to inhibit (via CYP3A4 inhibition) the inactivation or bioactivation of ritonavir in human liver microsomes; thus, the drug combination can effectively boost lopinavir concentrations. On the other hand, experiments in primary human hepatocytes indicated that lopinavir, in contrast to ritonavir (see above), had little inductive effects toward metabolism enzymes, although more systematic studies are needed to confirm this (lack of induction property) characteristic.

4.4   Fusion Inhibitors

4.4.1   Enfuvirtide

Enfuvirtide is not metabolized by CYP450 or UGT enzymes in humans. Based on these properties, it is not likely to be subject to metabolism-mediated drug-drug interactions. These properties are confirmed in patients [37], which will be discussed in separate chapters in this book.

4.5   Entry Inhibitors

4.5.1   Maraviroc

Maraviroc is oxidized and glucuronidated into various metabolites in humans. The primary enzymes responsible for the N-dealkylation of maraviroc are CYP3A4 and CYP3A5. This was based on the observation that CYP3A4 exhibited the highest catalytic activity in the oxidation of maraviroc in a panel of cDNA-expressed CYP450 enzymes and that ketoconazole (at inhibitory concentrations selective for CYP3A4) significantly reduced the metabolism of maraviroc in human liver microsomes [38]. CYP3A5 may play a more prominent role in maraviroc metabolism than CYP3A4 because liver microsomes from donors known to carry polymorphic CYP3A5*3 allele (loss of catalytic activity) exhibited significantly reduced N-dealkylated metabolite formation in the incubation medium compared to microsomes obtained from wild-type individuals [39]. Little is known about the specific

UGT enzymes responsible for the glucuronidation or the inhibition/induction potential of maraviroc in humans.

4.6   Integrase Inhibitors

4.6.1   Dolutegravir

Dolutegravir is primarily conjugated by UGT1A1 and CYP3A4 in humans. This was demonstrated in a panel of cDNA-expressed UGTs and CYPs where these two enzymes were the primary catalysts for dolutegravir metabolism [40]. Chemical inhibition experiments indicated that atazanavir (as UGT1A1-selective inhibitor) and azamulin (as CYP3A4-selective inhibitor) were able to significantly reduce the oxidative metabolism and conjugation of dolutegravir, respectively. In human liver microsomes, dolutegravir did not inhibit the metabolism of marker substrates for a variety of CYP, UGT, and transporters. Likewise, little induction of mRNAs for CYP1A2, CYP2B6, or CYP3A4 was observed in primary human hepatocytes, confirming the minimal drug-interaction potential of dolutegravir in general.

4.6.2   Elvitegravir

Elvitegravir is primarily metabolized by CYP3A4, UGT1A1, and UGT1A3 in humans as reported by the manufacturer (little information on their methodology disclosed); thus, it may be subject to drug-drug interactions mediated by these enzymes. To our knowledge, systematic investigations on the drug-interaction potentials for elvitegravir have not been conducted extensively in in vitro models.

4.6.3   Raltegravir

UGT1A1 is primarily responsible for the metabolism of raltegravir in humans. This was demonstrated in a panel of cDNA-expressed UGT enzymes where UGT1A1 was the primary catalyst and in human liver microsomes where bilirubin or B-estradiol (competitive inhibitors for UGT1A1) significantly inhibited the glucuronidation of raltegravir [41]. Despite some catalytic activity from cDNA-expressed UGT1A9, the activity of raltegravir glucuronidation did not correlate with that of propofol glucuronidation (marker reaction for UGT1A9), suggesting the lack of significant contribution from this enzyme. To our knowledge, drug-interaction potential for raltegravir using in vitro models has not been reported extensively in the literature.

4.7 Summary

Molecular drug-drug interactions mediated by CYP and UGT enzymes are commonly associated with NNRTIs, PIs, maraviroc, and integrase inhibitors, whereas the NRTIs and fusion inhibitor enfuvirtide are relatively inert because they are not cleared by these enzymes. Although specific antiretroviral agents can be subjected to metabolism by and exhibit modulatory effects toward a variety of CYP450 enzymes, the most common CYP450 enzyme involved in antiretroviral drug metabolism is CYP3A4, where the majority of NNRTIs are substrates/inducers and PIs tend to be substrate/inhibitors (with some induction effects evident for specific agents). As such, most of the drug-drug interactions observed in the clinic are expected to have resulted from these two classes of antiretroviral agents via the modulation of CYP3A4. On the other hand, the integrase inhibitors are known to be metabolized by UGT enzymes; thus, conjugation-associated drug interactions are more likely responsible for drug interactions linked to dolutegravir, elvitegravir, and raltegravir. However, compared to CYP450 enzymes, less is known about interactions mediated by UGT enzymes (due to lack of selective inhibitors and modulators); thus, more experiments are needed to characterize the drug interaction potential of these agents. As it stands, the current data likely underreport the number of drug interactions associated with the integrase inhibitors.

The majority of the data presented in this chapter are primarily obtained from molecular reaction phenotyping and drug inhibition studies using industry/regulatory body standardized approaches: cDNA-expressed enzymes, human liver microsomes, enzyme-selective chemical inhibitors, enzyme-specific monoclonal inhibitory antibodies, and correlational analyses. The majority of the studies have used a complement of these approaches; thus, the definitive drug metabolism enzyme(s) involved in these reactions can be identified. However, the majority of the data collected have focused only on the effects of a single modulator toward a single substrate, which may not be applicable to the clinical situation where polypharmacy incorporating multiple HIV drugs is commonly utilized. Hence, drug-drug interactions associated with combination enzyme modulators are needed in the in vitro setting as well. Likewise, relatively little information is known about the induction potential of the antiretroviral agents, which is more difficult to characterize due the need to utilize more complex in vitro systems such as primary cultures of human liver hepatocytes. As such, further in vitro studies are needed to elucidate the induction mechanism associated with various agents identified in this chapter.

References

1. Voorman RL, Maio SM, Hauer MJ, Sanders PE, Payne NA, Ackland MJ (1998) Metabolism of delavirdine, a human immunodeficiency virus type-1 reverse transcriptase inhibitor, by microsomal cytochrome P450 in humans, rats, and other species: probable involvement of CYP2D6 and CYP3A. Drug Metab Dispos 26(7):631–639

2. Voorman RL, Maio SM, Payne NA, Zhao Z, Koeplinger KA, Wang X (1998) Microsomal metabolism of delavirdine: evidence for mechanism-based inactivation of human cytochrome P450 3A. J Pharmacol Exp Ther 287(1):381–388

3. Voorman RL, Payne NA, Wienkers LC, Hauer MJ, Sanders PE (2001) Interaction of delavirdine with human liver microsomal cytochrome P450: inhibition of CYP2C9, CYP2C19, and CYP2D6. Drug Metab Dispos 29(1):41–47

4. Ward BA, Gorski JC, Jones DR, Hall SD, Flockhart DA, Desta Z (2003) The cytochrome P450 2B6 (CYP2B6) is the main catalyst of efavirenz primary and secondary metabolism: implication for HIV/AIDS therapy and utility of efavirenz as a substrate marker of CYP2B6 catalytic activity. J Pharmacol Exp Ther 306(1):287–300

5. Belanger AS, Caron P, Harvey M, Zimmerman PA, Mehlotra RK, Guillemette C (2009) Glucuronidation of the antiretroviral drug efavirenz by UGT2B7 and an in vitro investigation of drug-drug interaction with zidovudine. Drug Metab Dispos 37(9):1793–1796

6. Mugundu GM, Hariparsad N, Desai PB (2010) Impact of ritonavir, atazanavir and their combination on the CYP3A4 induction potential of efavirenz in primary human hepatocytes. Drug Metab Lett 4(1):45–50

7. Keubler A, Weiss J, Haefeli WE, Mikus G, Burhenne J (2012) Drug interaction of efavirenz and midazolam: efavirenz activates the CYP3A-mediated midazolam 1′-hydroxylation in vitro. Drug Metab Dispos 40(6):1178–1182

8. Ji HY, Lee H, Lim SR, Kim JH, Lee HS (2012) Effect of efavirenz on UDP-glucuronosyltransferase 1A1, 1A4, 1A6, and 1A9 activities in human liver microsomes. Molecules 17(1):851–860

9. Yanakakis LJ, Bumpus NN (2012) Biotransformation of the antiretroviral drug etravirine: metabolite identification, reaction phenotyping, and characterization of autoinduction of cytochrome P450-dependent metabolism. Drug Metab Dispos 40(4):803–814

10. Erickson DA, Mather G, Trager WF, Levy RH, Keirns JJ (1999) Characterization of the in vitro biotransformation of the HIV-1 reverse transcriptase inhibitor nevirapine by human hepatic cytochromes P-450. Drug Metab Dispos 27(12):1488–1495

11. Lade JM, Avery LB, Bumpus NN (2013) Human biotransformation of the nonnucleoside reverse transcriptase inhibitor rilpivirine and a cross-species metabolism comparison. Antimicrob Agents Chemother 57(10):5067–5079

12. Weiss J, Haefeli WE (2013) Potential of the novel antiretroviral drug rilpivirine to modulate the expression and function of drug transporters and drug-metabolising enzymes in vitro. Int J Antimicrob Agents 41(5):484–487

13. McDowell JA, Chittick GE, Ravitch JR, Polk RE, Kerkering TM, Stein DS (1999) Pharmacokinetics of [(14)C]abacavir, a human immunodeficiency virus type 1 (HIV-1) reverse transcriptase inhibitor, administered in a single oral dose to HIV-1-infected adults: a mass balance study. Antimicrob Agents Chemother 43(12):2855–2861

14. Piliero PJ (2004) Pharmacokinetic properties of nucleoside/nucleotide reverse transcriptase inhibitors. J Acquir Immune Defic Syndr 37(Suppl 1):S2–S12

15. Nekvindova J, Masek V, Veinlichova A, Anzenbacherova E, Anzenbacher P, Zidek Z et al (2006) Inhibition of human liver microsomal cytochrome P450 activities by adefovir and tenofovir. Xenobiotica 36(12):1165–1177

16. Barbier O, Turgeon D, Girard C, Green MD, Tephly TR, Hum DW et al (2000) 3′-azido-3′-deoxythimidine (AZT) is glucuronidated by human UDP-glucuronosyltransferase 2B7 (UGT2B7). Drug Metab Dispos 28(5):497–502

17. Trapnell CB, Klecker RW, Jamis-Dow C, Collins JM (1998) Glucuronidation of 3′-azido-3′-deoxythymidine (zidovudine) by human liver microsomes: relevance to clinical pharmacokinetic interactions with atovaquone, fluconazole, methadone, and valproic acid. Antimicrob Agents Chemother 42(7):1592–1596

18. Eagling VA, Howe JL, Barry MJ, Back DJ (1994) The metabolism of zidovudine by human liver microsomes in vitro: formation of 3′-amino-3′-deoxythymidine. Biochem Pharmacol 48(2):267–276

19. Pan-Zhou XR, Cretton-Scott E, Zhou XJ, Yang MX, Lasker JM, Sommadossi JP (1998) Role of human liver P450s and cytochrome b5 in the reductive metabolism of 3′-azido-3′-deoxythymidine (AZT) to 3′-amino-3′-deoxythymidine. Biochem Pharmacol 55(6):757–766

20. Zheng J (2002) Clinical pharmacology and biopharmaceutics review (21–567). Available at: http://www.accessdata.fda.gov/drugsatfda_docs/nda/2003/21-567_Reyataz_BioPharmr_P1.pdf. Accessed 6 June 2016

21. Arya V (2005) Clinical pharmacology and biopharmaceutics review (21–976). Available at: http://www.accessdata.fda.gov/drugsatfda_docs/nda/2006/021976s000_Sprycel_ClinPharmR.pdf. Accessed 6 June 2016

22. Decker CJ, Laitinen LM, Bridson GW, Raybuck SA, Tung RD, Chaturvedi PR (1998) Metabolism of amprenavir in liver microsomes: role of CYP3A4 inhibition for drug interactions. J Pharm Sci 87(7):803–807

23. von Moltke LL, Durol AL, Duan SX, Greenblatt DJ (2000) Potent mechanism-based inhibition of human CYP3A in vitro by amprenavir and ritonavir: comparison with ketoconazole. Eur J Clin Pharmacol 56(3):259–261

24. Chiba M, Hensleigh M, Nishime JA, Balani SK, Lin JH (1996) Role of cytochrome P450 3A4 in human metabolism of MK-639, a potent human immunodeficiency virus protease inhibitor. Drug Metab Dispos 24(3):307–314

25. Eagling VA, Back DJ, Barry MG (1997) Differential inhibition of cytochrome P450 isoforms by the protease inhibitors, ritonavir, saquinavir and indinavir. Br J Clin Pharmacol 44(2):190–194

26. Iribarne C, Berthou F, Carlhant D, Dreano Y, Picart D, Lohezic F et al (1998) Inhibition of methadone and buprenorphine N-dealkylations by three HIV-1 protease inhibitors. Drug Metab Dispos 26(3):257–260

27. Fayz S, Inaba T (1998) Zidovudine azido-reductase in human liver microsomes: activation by ethacrynic acid, dipyridamole, and indomethacin and inhibition by human immunodeficiency virus protease inhibitors. Antimicrob Agents Chemother 42(7):1654–1658

28. Ernest CS 2nd, Hall SD, Jones DR (2005) Mechanism-based inactivation of CYP3A by HIV protease inhibitors. J Pharmacol Exp Ther 312(2):583–591

29. Hirani VN, Raucy JL, Lasker JM (2004) Conversion of the HIV protease inhibitor nelfinavir to a bioactive metabolite by human liver CYP2C19. Drug Metab Dispos 32(12):1462–1467

30. Lillibridge JH, Liang BH, Kerr BM, Webber S, Quart B, Shetty BV et al (1998) Characterization of the selectivity and mechanism of human cytochrome P450 inhibition by the human immunodeficiency virus-protease inhibitor nelfinavir mesylate. Drug Metab Dispos 26(7):609–616

31. Kumar GN, Rodrigues AD, Buko AM, Denissen JF (1996) Cytochrome P450-mediated metabolism of the HIV-1 protease inhibitor ritonavir (ABT-538) in human liver microsomes. J Pharmacol Exp Ther 277(1):423–431

32. Liu L, Mugundu GM, Kirby BJ, Samineni D, Desai PB, Unadkat JD (2012) Quantification of human hepatocyte cytochrome P450 enzymes and transporters induced by HIV protease inhibitors using newly validated LC-MS/MS cocktail assays and RT-PCR. Biopharm Drug Dispos 33(4):207–217

33. Eagling VA, Wiltshire H, Whitcombe IW, Back DJ (2002) CYP3A4-mediated hepatic metabolism of the HIV-1 protease inhibitor saquinavir in vitro. Xenobiotica 32(1):1–17

34. Granfors MT, Wang JS, Kajosaari LI, Laitila J, Neuvonen PJ, Backman JT (2006) Differential inhibition of cytochrome P450 3A4, 3A5 and 3A7 by five human immunodeficiency virus (HIV) protease inhibitors in vitro. Basic Clin Pharmacol Toxicol 98(1):79–85

35. Rajagopalan P (2000) Clinical pharmacology and biopharmaceutics reviews (21–226). Available at: http://www.accessdata.fda.gov/drugsatfda_docs/nda/2000/21-226_Kaletra_biopharmr_P1.pdf. Accessed 6 June 2016

36. Weemhoff JL, von Moltke LL, Richert C, Hesse LM, Harmatz JS, Greenblatt DJ (2003) Apparent mechanism-based inhibition of human CYP3A in-vitro by lopinavir. J Pharm Pharmacol 55(3):381–386

37. Zhang X, Lalezari JP, Badley AD, Dorr A, Kolis SJ, Kinchelow T et al (2004) Assessment of drug-drug interaction potential of enfuvirtide in human immunodeficiency virus type 1-infected patients. Clin Pharmacol Ther 75(6):558–568

38. Hyland R, Dickins M, Collins C, Jones H, Jones B (2008) Maraviroc: in vitro assessment of drug-drug interaction potential. Br J Clin Pharmacol 66(4):498–507

39. Lu Y, Hendrix CW, Bumpus NN (2012) Cytochrome P450 3A5 plays a prominent role in the oxidative metabolism of the anti-human immunodeficiency virus drug maraviroc. Drug Metab Dispos 40(12):2221–2230

40. Reese MJ, Savina PM, Generaux GT, Tracey H, Humphreys JE, Kanaoka E et al (2013) In vitro investigations into the roles of drug transporters and metabolizing enzymes in the disposition and drug interactions of dolutegravir, a HIV integrase inhibitor. Drug Metab Dispos 41(2):353–361

41. Kassahun K, McIntosh I, Cui D, Hreniuk D, Merschman S, Lasseter K et al (2007) Metabolism and disposition in humans of raltegravir (MK-0518), an anti-AIDS drug targeting the human immunodeficiency virus 1 integrase enzyme. Drug Metab Dispos 35(9):1657–1663

Chapter 5
Clinical Drug-Drug Interaction Data: Effects of Co-administered Drugs on Pharmacokinetics of Antiretroviral Agents

Tony K.L. Kiang, Kyle John Wilby, and Mary H.H. Ensom

This chapter summarizes the clinical drug-drug interaction data for each antiretroviral agent. The effects of co-administered drugs on the pharmacokinetics of the following agents will be presented:

Nonnucleoside reverse transcriptase inhibitors (NNRTIs): delavirdine, efavirenz, etravirine, nevirapine, and rilpivirine

Nucleoside reverse-transcriptase inhibitors (NRTIs): abacavir, didanosine, and zidovudine

Protease inhibitors (PIs): atazanavir, darunavir, fosamprenavir, emtricitabine, lamivudine, stavudine, tenofovir, indinavir, nelfinavir, ritonavir, saquinavir, tipranavir, and lopinavir

Fusion Inhibitors: enfuvirtide

Entry inhibitors: maraviroc

Integrase inhibitors: dolutegravir, elvitegravir, raltegravir

Methodology: A systematic literature search on PubMed and Google Scholar was conducted, and the results cross-referenced with the prescribing information published by each manufacturer (as part of the FDA drug approval process) and Guidelines for the Use of Antiretroviral Agents in HIV-1-Infected Adults and Adolescent (AIDS info) published by the National Institutes of Health Research (Expert Guidelines) [1]. Only interactions supported by actual human data are presented in this chapter and theoretically possible interactions are omitted.

T.K.L. Kiang • M.H.H. Ensom (✉)
Faculty of Pharmaceutical Sciences, The University of British Columbia, Vancouver, BC, Canada
e-mail: tkiang@gmail.com; mary.ensom@ubc.ca

K.J. Wilby
College of Pharmacy, Qatar University, Doha, Qatar
e-mail: kjw@qu.edu.qa

© Springer Science+Business Media Singapore 2016   43
T.K.L. Kiang et al. (eds.), *Pharmacokinetic and Pharmacodynamic Drug Interactions Associated with Antiretroviral Drugs*,
DOI 10.1007/978-981-10-2113-8_5

Table 5.1 Effects of co-administered drugs on the pharmacokinetics of delavirdine [2, 5, 7, 9–12]

Drug	Summary effects on pharmacokinetics	Reference
Buprenorphine	No change in AUC, Cmax, CL/F, and t1/2	McCance-Katz 2006
Clarithromycin	No change in AUC, Cmax, or Cmin	FDA document
Didanosine	↓ AUC (38%), ↓ Cmax (51%)	Morse 1997
Fluconazole	No change in AUC, Cmax, Cmin, CL/F, and t1/2	Borin 1997
Indinavir	No change in pharmacokinetic parameters	Ferry 1998
Nelfinavir	↓ AUC (31%), ↓ Cmax (27%), ↓ Cmin (31%)	FDA document (abstract)
Rifabutin	↓ Cmax (75%), ↓ Cmin (95%), ↑ CL/F (5×), and ↓ t1/2 (56%)	Borin 1997
Rifampin	↓ Cmax (92%), ↑ CL/F (27×), and ↓ t1/2 (60%)	Borin 1997
Saquinavir	No change in pharmacokinetic parameters	FDA document
Zidovudine	No change in pharmacokinetic parameters	FDA document

AUC area-under-the curve, *CL/F* apparent oral clearance, *Cmax* maximum concentration, *Cmin* minimum concentration, *t1/2* half-life

5.1 Nonnucleoside Reverse Transcriptase Inhibitors (NNRTIs)

5.1.1 *Delavirdine* (Table 5.1)

5.1.1.1 Analgesics

The effects of steady-state buprenorphine (14–20 mg) on the pharmacokinetics of delavirdine (600 mg orally twice daily) in healthy subjects have been determined by McCance-Katz et al. [2]. Buprenorphine did not affect the area-under-the curve (AUC), maximum concentration (Cmax), or minimum concentration (Cmin) of delavirdine. Despite an increase (180%) in the time needed to reach maximum concentration (tmax), the apparent oral clearance (CL/F) of delavirdine did not change (Table 5.1). Delavirdine is primarily metabolized by CYP3A4 and CYP2D6 [3], and buprenorphine has not been known to inhibit these enzymes (despite being a substrate for CY3A4) [4]. These findings suggest a dose change is likely not required for delavirdine when co-administered with buprenorphine, although this suggestion still needs confirmation in the real patient population.

5.1.1.2 Antimicrobials

The effects of various antimicrobials on the pharmacokinetics of delavirdine have been tested in humans. When clarithromycin (500 mg orally twice daily) was co-administered with delavirdine (300 mg orally twice daily) under steady-state conditions, little effects of clarithromycin on the AUC, Cmax, and Cmin of delavirdine were observed [5]. These findings contradict the known metabolic properties of clarithromycin (a potent CYP3A4 inhibitor) [6] and delavirdine (primarily metabolized by CYP3A4), but may also be false negative results due to the small sample size used in the experiment. The lack of information on other pharmacokinetic parameters such as CL/F and apparent volume of distribution (Vd/F) precludes further mechanistic identification of the apparent lack of interaction in this drug-drug pairing.

These findings are consistent with the results from an experiment where delavirdine (300 mg orally three times daily) was co-administered with a another moderate CYP3A4 inhibitor, fluconazole (400 mg orally once daily), under steady-state conditions in HIV-infected individuals ($N = 13$) [7]. In this study, fluconazole also did not change the AUC, Cmax, tmax, CL/F, and t1/2 of delavirdine, supporting a lack of pharmacokinetic interaction between these agents. These two studies seem to suggest that CYP3A4 inhibitors (e.g., clarithromycin and fluconazole) [8] have little effects on the pharmacokinetics of delavirdine in humans, but further studies using larger patient populations and/or additional prototypical CYP3A4 inhibitors are needed to confirm this hypothesis.

In contrast to the finding of lack of effects on the pharmacokinetics of delavirdine from the co-administration of CYP3A4 inhibitors, significant pharmacokinetic drug interactions have been observed with CYP3A4 inducers in humans. In HIV-infected subjects, under steady-state conditions, both rifabutin (300 mg orally once daily, $N = 12$) and rifampin (600 mg orally once daily, $N = 12$) significantly decreased the Cmax (75 % and 92 %, respectively), t1/2 (56 % and 60 %, respectively), and increased the CL/F (5× and 27×, respectively) of delavirdine. These findings support the notion that increased CYP3A4 activity from rifabutin or rifampin co-administration led to significantly increased intrinsic clearance of delavirdine [9, 10]. Even though rifabutin was relatively less effective an inducer compared to rifampin, the co-administration of delavirdine is still contraindicated for both drugs, regardless of their potency of interaction. These findings also suggest that other potent CYP3A4 inducers can likely alter the pharmacokinetics of delavirdine.

5.1.1.3 Miscellaneous Agents

Population pharmacokinetic studies conducted by the manufacturer also indicated potential interactions with fluoxetine (increased Cmin of delavirdine) and anticonvulsants such as phenytoin, phenobarbital, or carbamazepine (decreased Cmin of delavirdine) [5]. However, until further studies using direct cohort comparisons have been conducted, the clinical significance of these findings still remain to be confirmed.

5.1.1.4 Protease Inhibitors

Data are available on the effects of protease inhibitors (indinavir, nelfinavir, and saquinavir) on the pharmacokinetics of delavirdine in humans [5]. A single dose of indinavir (400, 600, or 800 mg) had little effects on the Cmax and AUC of steady-state delavirdine (400 mg orally three times daily) in healthy subjects ($N=15$) [11]. In contrast, nelfinavir was able to significantly decrease the Cmax (27 %), AUC (31 %), and Cmin (31 %) of delavirdine in subjects infected with HIV. On the other hand, saquinavir (administered 600 mg orally three times daily) also had little effects on the pharmacokinetics of delavirdine (400 mg orally three times daily) in healthy subjects ($N=30$). These mixed findings may be the result of both inhibitory and induction effects of protease inhibitors toward the metabolism of delavirdine.

5.1.1.5   Nucleoside Reverse Transcriptase Inhibitors

The effects of didanosine and zidovudine on the pharmacokinetics of delavirdine have been characterized in humans. Morse et al. [12] demonstrated that a single dose of didanosine (125–200 mg tablet) decreased the Cmax (51 %) and AUC (38 %) of delavirdine (400 mg), without affecting the exposure of N-dealkylated delavirdine (primary oxidative metabolite of delavirdine) in HIV-infected patients ($N=12$). The interaction is likely not metabolism-mediated as evident by the lack of known inhibitory/inducing effects of didanosine (Chap. 4) and by the exposure of the primary oxidative metabolite (N-dealkylated delavirdine) remaining unchanged (suggesting un-perturbed delavirdine intrinsic clearance). On the other hand, the observed interaction is likely absorption related, where buffered didanosine formulation altered the gastric pH, thereby reducing the absorption of delavirdine. Supporting this hypothesis, a pH-related absorption interaction has been demonstrated with the concurrent use of antacids, H2 antagonists, or proton pump inhibitors [5]; therefore, simply separating the administration of didanosine and delavirdine may minimize the physical interaction. On the other hand, steady-state zidovudine (200 mg orally three times daily) had no effects on the pharmacokinetic parameters of steady-state delavirdine (400 mg orally three times daily, $N=42$), reflecting the nonoverlapping metabolic characteristics of delavirdine (primarily metabolized by CYP3A4) and zidovudine (primarily conjugated by UGT enzymes) in humans (Chap. 4).

5.1.2   Efavirenz (Table 5.2)

5.1.2.1   Antimicrobials

The effects of several antimicrobial agents (azithromycin, clarithromycin, fluconazole, rifabutin, rifampin, and voriconazole) on the pharmacokinetics of efavirenz have been reported. For the macrolides, azithromycin given at a single dose (600 mg) did not affect the steady-state pharmacokinetics of efavirenz (400 mg orally daily, $N=14$) [13]. This is in contrast to the findings obtained with clarithromycin (500 mg

Table 5.2 Effects of co-administered drugs on the pharmacokinetics of efavirenz [13, 16, 17]

Drug	Summary effects on pharmacokinetics	Reference
Azithromycin	No change in pharmacokinetic parameters	FDA document
Carbamazepine	↓ AUC (36%), ↓ Cmax (21%)	Ji 2008
Clarithromycin	No change in AUC, ↑ Cmax (11%)	FDA document
Cetirizine	↓ AUC (8%)	FDA document
Darunavir/ritonavir	↑ AUC (21%), ↑ Cmin, Cmax (15–17%)	Sekar 2007
Ethinyl estradiol	No change in pharmacokinetic parameters	FDA document
Fluconazole	↑ AUC (16%), no change in Cmax	FDA document
Indinavir	No change in pharmacokinetic parameters	FDA document
Lopinavir/ritonavir	↓ AUC (16%), no change in Cmax	FDA document
Nelfinavir	No change in pharmacokinetic parameters	FDA document
Paroxetine	No change in pharmacokinetic parameters	FDA document
Rifabutin	No change in pharmacokinetic parameters	FDA document
Rifampin	↓ AUC (26%), ↓ Cmax (20%)	FDA document
Ritonavir	↑ AUC (21%), ↑ Cmax (14%)	FDA document
Saquinavir	↓ AUC (12%), ↓ Cmax (14%)	FDA document
Sertraline	No change in AUC, ↑ Cmax (11%)	FDA document
Voriconazole	↑ AUC (44%), ↑ Cmax (38%)	FDA document

AUC area-under-the curve, *Cmax* maximum concentration, *Cmin* minimum concentration

orally twice daily) which increased Cmax (11%), but not the AUC of efavirenz (400 mg orally daily), when both were administered under steady-state conditions [13]. These findings are consistent with the relatively more potent inhibitory effects of clarithromycin toward CYP3A4 (one of the primary enzymes responsible for the oxidation of efavirenz) than azithromycin [14]. However, despite the lack of change in efavirenz exposure from macrolide co-administrations, the inductive effects of efavirenz toward these agents should be considered when evaluating the combination of these agents (see Chap. 6).

Differential effects on efavirenz pharmacokinetics were observed from fluconazole and voriconazole [13]. Under steady-state conditions, fluconazole (200 mg orally daily) did not affect the Cmax and increased the AUC (16%) of efavirenz (400 mg orally daily, $N = 10$) only modestly. This is in contrast to significant elevations of efavirenz Cmax (38%) and AUC (44%) when voriconazole (400 mg orally every 12 h×1 day, then 200 mg every 12 h) was co-administered under steady-state conditions. The differences in the degrees of pharmacokinetic interactions correspond to the potency of CYP3A4 inhibition by fluconazole (moderate inhibitor) and voriconazole (potent inhibitor) [8]. These findings also suggest the use of fluconazole over voriconazole for patients taking efavirenz should an azole antifungal be needed for the treatment of infections.

The effects of CYP3A4 inducers on the pharmacokinetics of efavirenz have also been characterized in humans. Rifabutin (600 mg orally daily for 7 days) did not change the Cmax or AUC, whereas rifampin (600 mg orally daily for 7 days) significantly attenuated the Cmax (20%) and AUC (26%) of efavirenz (600 mg orally for 7 or 14 days, respectively, $N=11$–12). These findings confirm the relatively more potent inductive effects of rifampin toward the CYP3A4 enzyme, the primary catalyst for efavirenz oxidation (Chap. 4), than rifabutin [15]. Based on these results, in the scenario where an antitubercular agent is warranted, rifabutin should be used instead of rifampin to minimize the possibility of reduced efavirenz efficacy.

5.1.2.2   Miscellaneous Agents

The effects of carbamazepine, cetirizine, ethinyl estradiol, and paroxetine on the pharmacokinetics of efavirenz have been characterized in humans. In healthy subjects receiving steady-state efavirenz (600 mg orally daily) and carbamazepine (400 mg orally daily), the AUC (36%) and Cmax (21%) of efavirenz were significantly reduced [16]. The induction of CYP3A4 and/or CYP2B6 (the primary enzymes responsible for efavirenz metabolism) by carbamazepine is the proposed mechanism behind the interaction with efavirenz, although metabolite analysis to characterize altered intrinsic clearance is needed to confirm this hypothesis. Although it is unclear if altered pharmacokinetics would result in clinically significant reduction in efavirenz efficacy, these findings suggest that alternative antiseizure/pain pharmacotherapy other than carbamazepine should be considered when used in combination with efavirenz. On the other hand, single-dose cetirizine (10 mg), single dose ethinyl estradiol (50 µg), steady-state paroxetine (20 mg orally daily), and steady-state sertraline (50 mg orally daily) had very little effects on the exposure of steady-state efavirenz (400–600 mg orally daily) in humans ($N=12$–13) [13]. These findings are consistent with the metabolic properties of these drugs that lack interaction potential with the known metabolic pathways of efavirenz.

5.1.2.3   Protease Inhibitors

The effects of various protease inhibitors (darunavir, indinavir, lopinavir/ritonavir, nelfinavir, ritonavir, and saquinavir) on the pharmacokinetics of efavirenz have been characterized. In healthy subjects, steady-state darunavir/ritonavir (300 mg/100 mg orally twice daily) significantly increased the Cmax (17%) and AUC (21%) of efavirenz (600 mg orally daily) [17]. Ritonavir alone also had similar effects on efavirenz (600 mg orally daily) exposure (i.e., increased by 21%), but this was observed only at a higher dose of ritonavir (i.e., 500 mg orally every 12 h, steady-state conditions) [13]. Because both darunavir and ritonavir are known potent inhibitors for CYP3A4 [18, 19], it was not possible to determine, based on these experiments, the relative inhibitory effects of darunavir and ritonavir toward efavirenz metabolism. On the other hand, neither indinavir (800 mg orally three times daily) nor nelfinavir (750 mg orally three times daily) altered the pharmacokinetics of efavirenz (200 or 600 mg orally daily, respectively) under steady-state dosing conditions ($N=10$–11) [13]. This is contradictory to the known inhibitory effects of indinavir and nelfinavir toward CYP3A4 [20, 21], but may be explained by the relatively reduced potency of CYP3A inhibition by these two protease inhibitors (Ki ~0.2–0.3 μM) in comparison to ritonavir (Ki ~0.03 μM), as demonstrated in vitro in human liver microsomes [22]. These findings highlight the importance of such in vitro enzyme inhibition data, which may be utilized to interpret clinical drug-drug interaction findings.

In contrast to the mentioned inhibitors, both lopinavir/ritonavir and saquinavir appeared to increase the intrinsic clearance of efavirenz in humans [13]. Under steady-state conditions, lopinavir/ritonavir (400 mg/100 mg orally every 12 h) significantly decreased the AUC, whereas saquinavir (1200 mg orally every 8 h) significantly decreased both Cmax (13 %) and AUC (12 %) of efavirenz (600 mg orally daily, $N = 11–13$). The effects of saquinavir may be explained by its known induction properties toward various CYP450 enzymes [23], which may have suppressed its own inhibitory effects toward CYP3A4 (main enzyme for the metabolism of efavirenz), resulting in a net enzyme induction effect. On the other hand, lopinavir is not known to have induction properties (Chap. 4); thus, the apparent induction effect from the lopinavir/ritonavir combination may be the action of ritonavir, which is known to induce a wide spectrum of CYP450 enzymes, including CYP2B6 which is also responsible for efavirenz oxidation (Chap. 4).

5.1.3   *Etravirine* (Table 5.3)

5.1.3.1   Antimalarial

The effects of a 3-day treatment course of artemether/lumefantrine (80 mg/480 mg) on the pharmacokinetics of steady-state etravirine (200 mg orally twice daily) were determined in healthy subjects ($N = 33$) [24]. Artemether/lumefantrine did not change the exposure of etravirine, which corresponded to the lack of adverse effects associated with the co-administration. Despite the fact that artemether/lumefantrine and etravirine are metabolized by CYP3A4, these data suggest that artemether/lumefantrine had little inhibitory effects toward this enzyme. Because etravirine is able to reduce the exposure of artemether/lumefantrine (Chap. 6), the co-administration of these agents is still not recommended.

5.1.3.2   Antimicrobials

The effects of several antimicrobial agents (clarithromycin, fluconazole, rifabutin, and voriconazole) on the pharmacokinetics of etravirine have been reported. With respect to drugs known to inhibit CYP450 enzymes, clarithromycin given at 500 mg twice daily increased Cmax (46 %) and AUC (42 %) of etravirine [25]. Similar effects on efavirenz pharmacokinetics were also observed from both fluconazole and voriconazole co-administration [26], where fluconazole and

Table 5.3 Effects of co-administered drugs on the pharmacokinetics of etravirine [24–26]

Drug	Summary effects on pharmacokinetics	Reference
Artemether/lumefantrine	No change in pharmacokinetic parameters	Kakuda 2013
Atazanavir	↑ AUC (50%), ↑ Cmax (47%)	FDA document
Atazanavir/ritonavir	↑ AUC (30%), ↑ Cmin (30%)	FDA document
Atorvastatin	No change in pharmacokinetic parameters	FDA document
Boceprevir	↓ AUC (23%), ↓ Cmax (24%)	Hammond 2013
Clarithromycin	↑ AUC (42%), ↑ Cmax (46%)	FDA document
Darunavir/ritonavir	↓ AUC (37%), ↓ Cmin (49%)	FDA document
Didanosine	No change in pharmacokinetic parameters	FDA document
Fluconazole	↑ AUC (86%)	Kakuda 2013
Lopinavir/ritonavir	No change in pharmacokinetic parameters	FDA document
Omeprazole	↑ AUC (41%)	FDA document
Paroxetine	No change in pharmacokinetic parameters	FDA document
Rifabutin	↓ AUC (37%), ↓ Cmax (37%)	FDA document
Raltegravir	No change in pharmacokinetic parameters	FDA document
Ritonavir	↑ AUC (17%), ↑ Cmax (15%)	FDA document
Saquinavir/ritonavir	↓ AUC (33%), ↓ Cmax (37%)	FDA document
Tenofovir	↓ AUC Cmax (19%)	FDA document
Tipranavir/ritonavir	↓ AUC (76%), ↓ Cmax (71%)	FDA document
Voriconazole	↑ AUC (36%)	Kakuda 2013

AUC area-under-the curve, *Cmax* maximum concentration, *Cmin* minimum concentration

voriconazole (200 mg orally daily) both increased the AUC (86% and 36%, respectively) of etravirine under steady-state conditions in healthy volunteers ($N = 18$). These findings are in agreement with the metabolic characteristics of clarithromycin, fluconazole, voriconazole (inhibitors of CYP3A4), and etravirine (a substrate of CYP3A4) [27]. The higher etravirine AUC from fluconazole administration compared to voriconazole is inconsistent with the known relative potency typically exhibited by these agents (voriconazole being a more potent inhibitor). Nevertheless, these results suggest that the co-administration of these agents should be avoided. On the other hand, the effects of a CYP3A4 inducer on the pharmacokinetics of etravirine have also been characterized in humans, where rifabutin (300 mg orally daily) significantly decreased the Cmax (27%) and AUC (27%) of etravirine ($N = 12$). It is not clear whether the relatively small magnitude of AUC change from rifabutin may be clinically significant, and one might hypothesize that rifampin (data not available) would likely lead to a bigger induction effect compared to rifabutin. These findings are consistent with the metabolic characteristics of rifabutin (inducer of CYP3A4) and etravirine (a substrate of CYP3A4).

5.1.3.3 Miscellaneous Agents

The effects of atorvastatin, omeprazole, paroxetine, and boceprevir on the pharmacokinetics of etravirine have been characterized in humans. Atorvastatin (40 mg orally daily) and paroxetine (20 mg orally daily) did not change the pharmacokinetics, whereas omeprazole and boceprevir both significantly increased the Cmax (17% and 24%, respectively) and AUC (41% and 23%, respectively) of etravirine [25, 28]. These findings are consistent with the metabolic properties of atorvastatin and paroxetine, as neither is known to be a strong inhibitor of CYP3A4 or CYP2C19, which are the primary enzymes responsible for etravirine metabolism (Chap. 4). In contrast, the inhibition by omeprazole of CYP2C19 [29] and boceprevir of CYP3A4 [30] is the likely mechanism associated with the increased exposure of etravirine in these studies.

5.1.3.4 Protease Inhibitors

Mixed effects of various protease inhibitors (atazanavir, atazanavir/ritonavir, darunavir/ritonavir, lopinavir/ritonavir, ritonavir, and saquinavir/ritonavir, and tipranavir/ritonavir) on the pharmacokinetics of efavirenz have been characterized. Atazanavir (400 mg orally daily), atazanavir/ritonavir (300 mg/100 mg daily), and lopinavir/ritonavir (400 mg/100 mg twice daily) increased the AUC (50%, 30%, 17% [nonsignificant elevation], respectively) and Cmax (47%, 30%, and 15% [nonsignificant elevation], respectively) of etravirine in humans [25]. On the other hand, darunavir/ritonavir (600 mg/100 mg twice daily), ritonavir (600 mg twice daily), saquinavir/ritonavir (1000 mg/100 mg twice daily), and tipranavir/ritonavir (500 mg/200 mg twice daily) significantly decreased the AUC (27%, 46%, 33%, 76%, respectively) and Cmax (32%, 32%, 37%, 71%, respectively) of etravirine. The apparent increased etravirine exposure from the co-administration of atazanavir, atazanavir/ritonavir, and lopinavir may be explained by their inhibitory effects toward CYP3A4 [31], one of the primary enzymes responsible for the oxidation of etravirine (Chap. 4). In contrast, it is not clear, based on the known metabolic properties, how darunavir/ritonavir, ritonavir, saquinavir/ritonavir, and tipranavir/ritonavir decrease the exposure of etravirine. Darunavir is known to be a potent inhibitor of CYP3A4, but little is known of its induction potential (Chap. 4). Because both ritonavir and saquinavir are capable of inhibiting and inducing CYP450 enzymes, their effects (when ritonavir is used in combination to boost the effects of other protease inhibitors) might be a summation of these opposing interacting activities. Further mechanistic studies are required to elucidate the exact interacting mechanisms.

5.1.3.5 Nucleoside Reverse Transcriptase Inhibitors and Integrase Inhibitors

The ability of didanosine (400 mg orally daily), tenofovir disoproxil fumarate (300 mg orally daily), and raltegravir (400 mg orally twice daily) to alter the pharmacokinetics of etravirine has been characterized in humans [25]. Except for the moderate decrease in etravirine AUC (21 %), no significant interactions by didanosine and raltegravir on the exposure of etravirine were observed. These data are supported by the general lack of metabolism-mediated drug interaction potential of didanosine (Chap. 4) and the nonoverlapping metabolic pathways between raltegravir (primarily metabolized by UGT enzymes, Chap. 4) and etravirine (CYP450 enzymes). Tenofovir has been primarily characterized as a nonpotent inhibitor of CYP450 enzymes (Chap. 4); thus, the apparent reduction of etravirine exposure, which may suggest an induction interaction, is not consistent with the known metabolic characteristics of these drugs. It is also unclear if the pharmacokinetic interaction, which appears to be moderate, would translate to pharmacodynamic alterations (e.g., decreased efficacy) of tenofovir.

5.1.4 Nevirapine (Table 5.4)

The effects of co-administered drugs on the pharmacokinetics of nevirapine have not been well characterized. In observational studies (data compared to historical controls), fluconazole (CYP3A4 inhibitor) was documented to increase nevirapine exposure by ~100 %, whereas rifampin (prototypical CYP3A4 inducer) decreased nevirapine exposure by ~50 % in HIV-infected individuals [32]. Although these experiments were not adequately controlled, they support the known fact that nevirapine is a substrate of CYP3A4 (Chap. 4). On the other hand, little effects of co-administered drugs (listed in Table 6.4: "Effects of nevirapine on the pharmacokinetics of co-administered drugs", Chap. 6) have been documented on the pharmacokinetics of nevirapine.

5.1.5 Rilpivirine (Table 5.5)

The effects of co-administered drugs on the pharmacokinetics of rilpivirine have been characterized extensively by the manufacturer, but these experiments were conducted at relatively higher concentrations of rilpivirine (i.e., 75 or 150 mg once daily), which have not been approved for therapeutic use (Table 5.5) [33]. As a result, these data would likely not be relevant for the clinic. On the other hand,

Table 5.4 Effects of co-administered drugs on the pharmacokinetics of nevirapine [32]

Drug	Summary effects on pharmacokinetics	Reference
Fluconazole	↑ AUC (100 %) vs. historical control	FDA document
Rifampin	↓ AUC (50 %) vs. historical control	FDA document

AUC area-under-the curve

Table 5.5 Effects of co-administered drugs on the pharmacokinetics of rilpivirine [33]

Drug	Summary effects on pharmacokinetics	Reference
Acetaminophen	↑ AUC (16%), ↑ Cmax (9%)	FDA document
Atorvastatin	↓ AUC (10%)	FDA document
Chlorzoxazone	↑ AUC (25%), ↑ Cmax (17%)	FDA document
Darunavir/ritonavir	↑ AUC (130%), ↑ Cmax (79%)	FDA document
Didanosine	No significant changes in pharmacokinetic parameters	FDA document
Ethinyl estradiol/ norethindrone	No significant changes in pharmacokinetic parameters (vs. historical control)	FDA document
Famotidine	↓ AUC (76%), ↓ Cmax (85%) – taken 2 h before ↑ AUC (13%), ↑ Cmax (21%) – taken 4 h after	FDA document
Lopinavir/ritonavir	↑ AUC (52%), ↑ Cmax (29%)	FDA document
Ketoconazole	↑ AUC (49%), ↑ Cmax (30%)	
Methadone	No significant changes in pharmacokinetic parameters (vs. historical control)	FDA document
Omeprazole	↓ AUC (40%), ↓ Cmin (33%)	FDA document
Rifabutin	↓ AUC (46%), ↓ Cmax (35%)	FDA document
Rifampin	↓ AUC (80%), ↓ Cmax (69%)	FDA document
Sildenafil	No significant changes in pharmacokinetic parameters	FDA document
Tenofovir	No significant changes in pharmacokinetic parameters	FDA document

Most of the drug interaction studies summarized in this table have been conducted at suprathera-peutic dosing of rilpivirine and may not be clinically relevant (see text for details)
AUC area-under-the curve, *Cmax* maximum concentration, *Cmin* minimum concentration

experiments testing the effects of steady-state ethinyl estradiol/norethindrone (0.035 mg/1 mg daily) or methadone (60–100 mg daily) on the pharmacokinetics of steady-state rilpivirine (approved dosing of 25 mg daily) have provided negative findings, although it is difficult to interpret these results because the experiments used historical cohorts for comparison. Based on these limitations, little is currently known about the clinical pharmacokinetic interactions associated with rilpivirine; however, because rilpivirine is primarily metabolized by CYP3A4 and UGT1A [34], it can potentially be subject to drug interactions mediated by these enzyme systems.

5.2 Nucleoside Reverse-Transcriptase Inhibitors (NRTIs)

5.2.1 *Abacavir* (Table 5.6)

Little information is available in the literature on metabolism-mediated drug-drug interactions associated with abacavir in humans, which is consistent with the fact that it is not a substrate of the CYP450 enzymes (Chap. 4). However, abacavir undergoes conjugation by UGTs (the exact identities of the enzymes involved remain to be determined) [35]; thus, its pharmacokinetics may be affected by modulators of phase II enzymes.

5.2.2   *Didanosine* (Table 5.7)

Very few metabolism-mediated drug-drug interaction studies have been published for didanosine, which is not known to be metabolized by CYP450, UGT, or transporter enzymes (Chap. 4). Because it undergoes purine-like metabolism in humans, drugs such as allopurinol and tenofovir can potentially increase its plasma concentration. This has been demonstrated in four HIV-infected subjects where the exposure of didanosine remained stable even when the dose of didanosine was halved in the presence of allopurinol (compared to the exposure values obtained from regular

Table 5.6 Effects of co-administered drugs on the pharmacokinetics of abacavir

Drug	Summary effects on pharmacokinetics	Reference
Limited published studies are available characterizing metabolism-mediated drug interactions associated with abacavir		

Table 5.7 Effects of co-administered drugs on the pharmacokinetics of didanosine [36, 37, 44]

Drug	Summary effects on pharmacokinetics	Reference
Allopurinol	↑ AUC (100%)	Boelaert 2002
Buprenorphine	No significant change in pharmacokinetic parameters	Baker 2010
Ganciclovir	↑ AUC (111%)	FDA document
Indinavir	No significant change in pharmacokinetic parameters	FDA document
Ketoconazole	No significant change in pharmacokinetic parameters	FDA document
Metoclopramide	↑ Cmax (13%)	FDA document
Ranitidine	↑ AUC (14%), ↑ Cmax (13%)	FDA document
Rifabutin	↑ AUC (13%), ↑ Cmax (17%)	FDA document
Ritonavir	↓ AUC (13%), ↓ Cmax (16%)	FDA document
Stavudine	No significant change in pharmacokinetic parameters	FDA document
Sulfamethoxazole	No significant change in pharmacokinetic parameters	FDA document
Tenofovir	↑ AUC (44%), ↑ Cmax (28%)	FDA document
Trimethoprim	No significant change in pharmacokinetic parameters	FDA document
Zidovudine	No significant change in pharmacokinetic parameters	FDA document

AUC area-under-the curve, *Cmax* maximum concentration

dosing of didanosine in the absence of allopurinol) [36]. Likewise, tenofovir diso-proxil fumarate (300 mg daily) was able to significantly increase the AUC and Cmax of didanosine (400 mg daily, in buffered solution) under steady-state conditions [37]. The proposed mechanism of interaction is the inhibition of purine nucleoside phosphorylase by allopurinol and tenofovir, an effect demonstrated in human T-leukemic CCRF-CEM lymphoblasts [38]. Based on these findings, the concurrent administration of didanosine with allopurinol is not recommended.

The majority of other tested drugs showed little effects on the pharmacokinetics of didanosine (Table 5.7) because there is no pharmacological basis to support these drug-drug interactions. Moreover, those experiments that did generate statistically significant interactions (e.g., ranitidine, Table 5.7) usually exhibited relatively small changes (~10%), which may be due to the small sample sizes and large variabilities found in the experiments [37]. The overall effects (if any) are not likely clinically significant.

5.2.3 *Emtricitabine* (Table 5.8)

Little information is available in the literature on drug-drug interactions associated with emtricitabine in humans, which may be due to the lack of a pharmacological basis for metabolism-related interactions associated with emtricitabine in general (Chap. 4). The manufacturer has conducted standard testing to determine the effects of various antivirals (famciclovir, indinavir, tenofovir, stavudine, and zidovudine) on the pharmacokinetics of emtricitabine (200 mg as single dose or steady-state conditions) [39] in healthy volunteers (Table 5.8), but none reported a significant effect.

5.2.4 *Lamivudine* (Table 5.9)

Little data have been published describing the drug-drug interactions associated with lamivudine in humans (Table 5.9). This is consistent with the lack of pharmacological basis for metabolism-related interactions associated with lamivudine in general (Chap. 4). In HIV-infected patients ($N = 12$) taking zidovudine (200 mg single dose), the pharmacokinetics of lamivudine (steady-state dosing, 300 mg every 12 h) did not change [40]. Similar observation of lack of pharmacokinetic interaction was also observed between lamivudine and interferon alpha in healthy volunteers ($N = 19$) [40]. On the other hand, trimethoprim/sulfamethoxazole (160 mg/800 mg daily) significantly increased the AUC (44%) of lamivudine (300 mg every 12 h) in HIV-infected patients ($N = 14$) under steady-state conditions, which corresponded with significantly reduced oral clearance (29%) and renal clearance (30%) of lamivudine. These data support the inhibition of renal tubular secretion by trimethoprim/sulfamethoxazole as the likely mechanism mediating the interaction associated with lamivudine. As a result, co-administration with trimethoprim/sulfamethoxazole is not recommended.

Table 5.8 Effects of co-administered drugs on the pharmacokinetics of emtricitabine [39]

Drug	Summary effects on pharmacokinetics	Reference
Famciclovir	No significant change in pharmacokinetic parameters	FDA document
Indinavir	No significant change in pharmacokinetic parameters	FDA document
Tenofovir	No significant change in pharmacokinetic parameters	FDA document
Stavudine	No significant change in pharmacokinetic parameters	FDA document
Zidovudine	No significant change in pharmacokinetic parameters	FDA document

Table 5.9 Effects of co-administered drugs on the pharmacokinetics of lamivudine [40]

Drug	Summary effects on pharmacokinetics	Reference
Interferon alpha	No significant change in pharmacokinetic parameters	FDA document
Trimethoprim/ sulfamethoxazole	↑ AUC (44 %), ↓ CL/F (29 %), ↓ renal clearance (30 %)	FDA document
Zidovudine	No significant change in pharmacokinetic parameters	FDA document

AUC area-under-the curve, *CL/F* apparent oral clearance

5.2.5 *Stavudine* (Table 5.10)

Little information is available in the literature on drug-drug interactions associated with stavudine in humans. This is supported by the lack of pharmacological basis for metabolism-related interactions associated with stavudine in general (Chap. 4). In HIV-infected subjects, didanosine (100 mg every 12 h×4 days), lamivudine (150 mg as single dose), and nelfinavir (750 mg every 8 h, steady-state conditions) did not affect the AUC of stavudine (40 mg as single dose or continuous dosing, $N=8$–18) [41]. On the other hand, opioid-dependent subjects ($N=17$) on stable methadone therapy exhibited decreased AUC (23 %) and Cmax (44 %) of stavudine compared to untreated controls, an effect likely associated with reduced stavudine absorption and not metabolism [42]. The clinical relevance of the methadone-stavudine interaction remains to be determined.

5.2.6 *Tenofovir* (Table 5.11)

Little literature has been published describing the drug-drug interactions associated with tenofovir in humans (Table 5.11). With the exception of atazanavir and lopinavir/ritonavir, none of the tested agents have produced a significant change in the

Table 5.10 Effects of co-administered drugs on the pharmacokinetics of stavudine [41, 42]

Drug	Summary effects on pharmacokinetics	Reference
Didanosine	No change in AUC, ↑ Cmax (17 %)	FDA document
Lamivudine	No change in AUC, ↑ Cmax (12 %)	FDA document
Methadone	↓AUC (23 %), ↓ Cmax (44 %)	Rainey 2000
Nelfinavir	No significant changes in pharmacokinetic parameters	FDA document

AUC area-under-the curve, *Cmax* maximum concentration

Table 5.11 Effects of co-administered drugs on the pharmacokinetics of tenofovir [43–45]

Drug	Summary effects on pharmacokinetics	Reference
Abacavir	No significant change in pharmacokinetic parameters	FDA document
Atazanavir	↑ AUC (24 %), ↑ Cmax (14 %)	FDA document
Buprenorphine	No significant change in pharmacokinetic parameters	Baker 2010
Didanosine	No significant change in pharmacokinetic parameters	FDA document
Emtricitabine	No significant change in pharmacokinetic parameters	FDA document
Entecavir	No significant change in pharmacokinetic parameters	FDA document
Indinavir	No significant change in pharmacokinetic parameters	FDA document
Lamivudine	No significant change in pharmacokinetic parameters	FDA document
Lopinavir/ritonavir	↑ AUC (32 %)	FDA document
Raltegravir	No significant change in pharmacokinetic parameters	Wenning 2008
Saquinavir/ritonavir	No significant change in pharmacokinetic parameters	FDA document

AUC area-under-the curve, *Cmax* maximum concentration

pharmacokinetics of tenofovir (Table 5.11) [43–45]. This is consistent with the lack of pharmacological basis for metabolism-related interactions associated with tenofovir in general (Chap. 4) (Table 5.11). Atazanavir (400 mg daily, $N=33$) and lopinavir/ritonavir (400 mg/100 mg daily, $N=24$) increased the AUC of tenofovir (300 mg daily) 24 % and 32 %, respectively, under steady-state conditions. However, the mechanisms associated with these significant findings could not be derived from the known metabolic characteristics of the drugs involved. It also remains to be determined if the relatively modest increases in tenofovir AUC would result in increased toxicity; therefore, close monitoring is suggested when the combination is administered.

5.2.7   *Zidovudine* (Table 5.12)

Zidovudine is primarily conjugated by UGT enzymes [46] and can be subject to drug-drug interactions mediated by UGT2B7 [47, 48]. Atovaquone (750 mg every 12 h, $N=14$), fluconazole (400 mg daily, $N=12$), lamivudine (300 mg every 12 h, $N=12$), methadone (30–90 mg daily, $N=9$), probenecid (500 mg every 6 h, $N=3$), and valproic acid (250–500 mg every 8 h, $N=6$) significantly increased the AUC (31 %, 74 %, 13 %, 43 %, 106 %, 80 %, respectively) of zidovudine under steady-state conditions in humans (Table 5.12). With the exception of lamivudine, all of these co-administered drugs are known to inhibit UGT enzymes [47, 49–52]. The effects of lamivudine on the exposure of zidovudine are relatively small (13 %) and has little pharmacological basis, based on known metabolism characteristics of either drug. These findings are also consistent with the data collected *in vitro*, where atovaquone, fluconazole, methadone, and valproic acid exhibited significant inhibitory activities toward the conjugation of zidovudine [47]. On the other hand, nelfinavir (750 mg every 8 h, $N=11$), rifampin (600 mg daily, $N=8$), and ritonavir (300 mg every 6 h, $N=9$) decreased the AUC of zidovudine by 35 %, 47 %, and 25 %, respectively, under steady-state conditions (Table 5.12) [53, 54]. Both rifampin and ritonavir have been known to induce UGT enzymes [54, 55], which is the likely mechanism responsible for the observed interaction. The effects of nelfinavir on the exposure of zidovudine cannot be explained by the known metabolism characteristics of either drug (Chap. 4).

5.3   Protease Inhibitors

5.3.1   *Atazanavir* (Table 5.13)

5.3.1.1   Antivirals

The effects of co-administered NNRTIs and NRTIs on the pharmacokinetics of individual protease inhibitors have been described in detail in other sections. Please refer to each individual table for details.

Table 5.12 Effects of co-administered drugs on the pharmacokinetics of zidovudine [53, 54]

Drug	Summary effects on pharmacokinetics	Reference
Atovaquone	↑ AUC (31 %)	FDA document
Fluconazole	↑ AUC (74 %)	FDA document
Lamivudine	↑ AUC (13 %)	FDA document
Methadone	↑ AUC (43 %)	FDA document
Nelfinavir	↓ AUC (35 %)	FDA document
Probenecid	↑ AUC (106 %)	FDA document
Rifampin	↓ AUC (47 %)	Gallicano 1999
Ritonavir	↓ AUC (25 %)	FDA document
Valproic acid	↑ AUC (80 %)	FDA document

AUC area-under-the curve

Table 5.13 Effects of co-administered drugs on the pharmacokinetics of atazanavir [56–58, 60]

Drug	Summary effects on pharmacokinetics	Reference
Atenolol	No significant changes in pharmacokinetic parameters	FDA document
Boceprevir	↓ AUC (35%)	Hulskotte 2013
Clarithromycin	↑ AUC (28%), no change in Cmax	FDA document
Diltiazem	No significant changes in pharmacokinetic parameters	FDA document
Famotidine	↓ AUC (up to 41%)	FDA document
Fluconazole	No significant changes in pharmacokinetic parameters	FDA document
Ketoconazole	No significant changes in pharmacokinetic parameters	FDA document
Omeprazole	↓ AUC (up to 94%)	FDA document
Posaconazole	↑ AUC (160%), ↑ Cmax (270%)	Krishna 2009
Rifabutin	No change in AUC, ↑ Cmax (34%)	FDA document
Rifampin	↓ AUC (72%), ↓ Cmax (53%)	FDA document
Ritonavir	↑ AUC (238%), ↑ Cmax (86%)	FDA document

AUC area-under-the curve, *Cmax* maximum concentration

The pharmacokinetic interaction between the hepatitis C protease inhibitor, boceprevir, and atazanavir has been characterized in healthy subjects ($N = 39$) [56]. Boceprevir (800 mg three times daily) significantly reduced the AUC of atazanavir (300 mg daily, boosted by ritonavir 100 mg) by 35%, but this pharmacokinetic interaction was not related to altered pharmacodynamic effects. The effects of the interaction between boceprevir (a CYP3A4 inhibitor) [30] and atazanavir (a CYP3A4 substrate) [57] are inconsistent with the known metabolic characteristics of either drug, suggesting alternative mechanisms may be involved. Based on the significant pharmacokinetic alteration observed, the co-administration of these agents is not recommended.

When ritonavir (100 mg daily, $N = 28$) is co-administered with atazanavir (300 mg daily), the AUC and Cmax of atazanavir were increased significantly by 238% and 86%, respectively, when compared to historical data using atazanavir alone [58]. Although this combination is not administered clinically, this experiment demonstrated the potent inhibitory effects of ritonavir toward CYP3A4. It also demonstrates that other prototypical inhibitors of this enzyme will likely have a significant pharmacokinetic interaction with atazanavir in humans.

5.3.1.2 Cardiovascular Agents

The effects of atenolol and diltiazem on the pharmacokinetics of atazanavir have been characterized in humans [58], and neither atenolol (50 mg daily, $N = 19$) nor diltiazem (180 mg daily, $N = 30$) significantly altered the pharmacokinetics of atazanavir (400 mg daily) under steady-state conditions. Atazanavir is metabolized by CYP3A4 [58], which is not likely modulated by atenolol. On the other hand, diltiazem is an inhibitor of CYP3A4 [59]; thus, the lack of pharmacokinetic interaction between diltiazem and atazanavir is inconsistent with this metabolic property, but may be explained by the "moderate" potency of inhibition exhibited by diltiazem toward this enzyme. Despite the lack of effects of either agent on the pharmacokinetics of atazanavir, the co-administration of these agents is not recommended because atazanavir is capable of increasing the exposures of both atenolol and diltiazem (Chap. 6).

5.3.1.3   Acid Reducing Agents

The effects of an H2-antagonist (famotidine) and proton pump inhibitor (omeprazole) on the pharmacokinetics of atazanavir have been determined [58]. Both famotidine (40 mg twice daily, $N=45$) and omeprazole (40 mg once daily, $N=48$) significantly reduced the AUC of atazanavir by 41 % and 94 %, respectively. These effects are explained by the reduced solubility of atazanavir in a less acidic environment, resulting in reduced absorption of the antiviral agent. The degree of interaction also corresponded with the potency of acid suppression mediated by these agents (i.e. omeprazole greater than famotidine), and these effects can likely apply to the entire class of acid reducing drugs in general.

5.3.1.4   Antimicrobials

Studies investigating the effects of clarithromycin, fluconazole, ketoconazole, posaconazole, rifabutin, and rifampin on the pharmacokinetics of atazanavir are available [58, 60]. Clarithromycin (500 mg twice daily, $N=29$) modestly increased the AUC (28 %) of atazanavir (400 mg daily) under steady-state conditions, which can be explained by the inhibitory effects of clarithromycin toward CYP3A4 [61], the primary enzyme responsible for the oxidation of atazanavir (Chap. 4). In contrast, neither fluconazole (200 mg daily, $N=29$) nor ketoconazole (200 mg daily, $N=14$) affected the exposure of atazanavir, despite their known inhibitory activities toward CYP3A4. The fact that posaconazole (400 mg twice daily) was capable of increasing the AUC (3.7×) of atazanavir (300 mg daily) in healthy volunteers suggests that relatively more potent inhibitors of CYP3A4 (such as posaconazole) can still have significant effects on the pharmacokinetics of atazanavir. These findings also suggest that fluconazole or ketoconazole can be used if an azole antifungal needs to be used in combination with atazanavir.

Differential effects of CYP3A4 inducers on the pharmacokinetics of atazanavir are also evident from rifabutin and rifampin [58]. The relatively stronger CYP3A4 inducer, rifampin, significantly decreased the AUC (72 %) and Cmax (53 %) of atazanavir (300 mg daily boosted with ritonavir 100 mg) under steady-state conditions ($N=16$), but rifabutin, a weaker inducer (150 mg daily, $N=7$), had little effects. These findings suggest that rifabutin would be the drug of choice (instead of rifampin) when these agents are needed for patients taking atazanavir.

5.3.2 *Darunavir* (Table 5.14)

5.3.2.1 Antivirals

The effects of co-administered NNRTIs, NRTIs, entry inhibitors, and integrase inhibitors on the pharmacokinetics of darunavir have been described in detail in other sections. Please refer to each individual table for details.

The pharmacokinetic interactions between the hepatitis C protease inhibitors (boceprevir, simeprevir, and telaprevir) and darunavir have been characterized in humans [62]. Boceprevir (800 mg three times daily, $N=11$) and telaprevir (750 mg three times daily, $N=11$) significantly reduced the AUC of darunavir (600 mg daily, boosted by ritonavir 100 mg) by 44% and 40%, respectively, whereas simeprevir (50 mg daily) modestly increased the AUC (18%) of unboosted darunavir (800 mg daily, $N=25$). The apparent interactions between boceprevir, telaprevir (CYP3A4 inhibitor) [30, 63], and darunavir (a CYP3A4 substrate) [18] are inconsistent with the known metabolic characteristics of these drugs, suggesting alternative mechanisms, such as the enzyme induction/inhibition effects of the pharmacological booster ritonavir, may be involved. The effects of simeprevir on the pharmacokinetics of darunavir are difficult to explain based on known pharmacokinetic characteristics of either agent. The significant reductions of darunavir exposure from boceprevir and telaprevir indicate that their co-administration is not recommended.

Table 5.14 Effects of co-administered drugs on the pharmacokinetics of darunavir [62]

Drug	Summary effects on pharmacokinetics	Reference
Artemether/lumefantrine	No significant changes in pharmacokinetic parameters	FDA document
Boceprevir	↓ AUC (44%), ↓ Cmax (36%)	FDA document
Carbamazepine	No significant changes in pharmacokinetic parameters	FDA document
Clarithromycin	No significant changes in pharmacokinetic parameters	FDA document
Ketoconazole	↑AUC (42%), ↑ Cmax (21%)	FDA document
Omeprazole	No significant changes in pharmacokinetic parameters	FDA document
Paroxetine	No significant changes in pharmacokinetic parameters	FDA document
Rifabutin	↑ AUC (57%), ↑ Cmax (42%)	FDA document
Sertraline	No significant changes in pharmacokinetic parameters	FDA document
Simeprevir	↑ AUC (18%)	FDA document
Telaprevir	↓ AUC (40%), ↓ Cmax (40%)	FDA document

AUC area-under-the curve, *Cmax* maximum concentration

5.3.2.2 Antimicrobials

Studies investigating the effects of clarithromycin, ketoconazole, and rifabutin on the pharmacokinetics of darunavir are available [62]. Clarithromycin (500 mg twice daily, $N = 17$) did not affect the exposure of darunavir (400 mg daily boosted with ritonavir 100 mg) under steady-state conditions. On the other hand, both ketoconazole (200 mg daily, $N = 14$) and rifabutin (150 mg every other day, $N = 11$) increased the AUC of darunavir (400 or 600 mg boosted with ritonavir 100 mg) by 42 % and 57 %, respectively. The effects of ketoconazole on darunavir exposure can be explained by its inhibition of CYP3A4, the primary enzyme responsible for the oxidation of darunavir (Chap. 4). However, the lack of interaction between clarithromycin and darunavir is contradictory to the known inhibitory effects of clarithromycin toward CYP3A4 [61]. Likewise, the effects of rifabutin on increased exposure of darunavir also contradict the known induction effects of rifabutin toward CYP3A4 [15]. It is possible that these contradictory findings may be due to mixed enzyme induction/inhibition effects from the pharmacological booster ritonavir, which was co-administered with darunavir in these experiments. Given the extent of increased exposure, these data indicate that the co-administration of darunavir (boosted by ritonavir) and ketoconazole or rifabutin should be avoided.

5.3.2.3 Miscellaneous Agents

No significant effects on the pharmacokinetics of darunavir (400–600 mg boosted with 100 mg ritonavir) have been observed in human subjects administered artemether/lumefantrine (80 mg/400 mg for 6 doses, $N = 14$), carbamazepine (200 mg twice daily, $N = 16$), omeprazole (20 mg daily, $N = 16$), paroxetine (20 mg daily, $N = 16$), or sertraline (50 mg daily, $N = 13$) under steady-state conditions [62]. These findings are inconsistent with the known potent induction effects of carbamazepine [64] or the potential inhibitory effects of artemether/lumefantrine (by virtue of being a substrate) toward CYP3A4. Again, it is possible that these contradictory findings may be due to mixed enzyme induction/inhibition effects from the pharmacological booster ritonavir, which was co-administered with darunavir in these experiments. On the other hand, the lack of effects from the proton pump inhibitor (omeprazole) and antidepressants (paroxetine and sertraline) on the pharmacokinetics of darunavir is in line with their primary inhibitory effects toward the CYP2C enzymes, which are not known to metabolize darunavir. Despite the lack of effects by these drugs on the pharmacokinetics of darunavir (boosted with ritonavir), their co-administration is still contraindicated due to significant effects of darunavir (boosted with ritonavir) on the exposure of these agents (Chap. 6).

5.3.3   *Fosamprenavir* (Table 5.15)

Fosamprenavir is a prodrug that is rapidly hydrolyzed in the gut in the formation of the active drug, amprenavir (Chap. 4). The drug interactions discussed in this chapter pertain to the active moiety.

5.3.3.1   Antivirals

The effects of co-administered NNRTIs, NRTIs, entry inhibitors, and integrase inhibitors on the pharmacokinetics of amprenavir have been described in detail in other sections. Please refer to each individual table for details.

The pharmacokinetic interactions between protease inhibitors (atazanavir, indinavir, lopinavir/ritonavir, and saquinavir) and amprenavir (± ritonavir) have been characterized in humans [65]. In combinations involving amprenavir boosted with ritonavir, atazanavir (300 mg daily, $N=22$) did not change the pharmacokinetics of amprenavir (700 mg twice daily with 100 mg ritonavir), but lopinavir/ritonavir (400 mg/100 mg twice daily, $N=18$) significantly decreased the AUC (63%) and Cmax (58%) of amprenavir under steady-state conditions. Both atazanavir [65] and lopinavir are potent inhibitors of CYP3A4, the enzyme primarily responsible for the oxidation of amprenavir in humans [66]; thus, these data support the lopinavir/ritonavir-mediated inhibition of CYP3A4 that resulted in increased exposure of amprenavir. In contrast, the lack of effects of atazanavir on the pharmacokinetics of boosted-amprenavir is more difficult to explain, but it is again possible that mixed enzyme induction/inhibition effects from the pharmacological booster ritonavir may have confounded the observation. Further experiments are needed to test this hypothesis.

In combinations involving amprenavir not boosted with ritonavir, indinavir (800 mg three times daily, $N=9$) increased the AUC (33%) and Cmax (18%), whereas saquinavir (800 mg three times daily, $N=7$) significantly decreased the AUC (32%) and Cmax (32%) of amprenavir (700–800 mg three times daily) under steady-state conditions [65]. These findings are consistent with the known inhibitory effects of indinavir [67] and the mixed inhibition/induction effects of saquinavir [23] toward CYP3A4, the primary enzyme responsible for the metabolism of amprenavir in humans (Chap. 4). The significant pharmacokinetic interactions indicate that the co-administration of these agents (which are unlikely combinations in the clinic) should be avoided.

5.3.3.2   Antimicrobials

The effects of various antimicrobials (clarithromycin, ketoconazole, posaconazole, rifabutin, and rifampin) on the pharmacokinetics of amprenavir (± ritonavir) have been characterized [65, 68]. Clarithromycin (500 mg twice daily, $N=12$)

Table 5.15 Effects of co-administered drugs on the pharmacokinetics of amprenavir (± ritonavir) (unboosted combinations will be designated) [65, 68]

Drug	Summary effects on pharmacokinetics	Reference
Atazanavir	No significant changes in pharmacokinetic interactions	FDA document
Atorvastatin	↓ AUC (27%)- unboosted No change in pharmacokinetic parameters – boosted with ritonavir	FDA document
Clarithromycin	↑ AUC (18%), ↑ Cmax (15%) – unboosted	FDA document
Esomeprazole	No significant changes in pharmacokinetic interactions	FDA document
Ethinyl estradiol/norethindrone	No significant changes in pharmacokinetic interactions – unboosted	FDA document
Indinavir	↑ AUC (33%),↑ Cmax (18%) – unboosted	FDA document
Ketoconazole	No significant changes in pharmacokinetic interactions ↑ AUC (31%), ↓ Cmax (16%)-unboosted	FDA document
Lopinavir/ritonavir	↓ AUC (63%), ↓ Cmax (58%)	FDA document
Methadone	No significant changes in pharmacokinetic interactions ↓ AUC (30%),↓ Cmax (27%)-unboosted	FDA document
Phenytoin	↑ AUC (20%)	FDA document
Posaconazole	No significant changes in pharmacokinetic interactions	Bruggermann 2010
Rifabutin	↑ AUC (35%) ↓ AUC (15%) – unboosted	FDA document
Rifampin	↓ AUC (82%), ↓ Cmax (70%) –unboosted	FDA document
Saquinavir	↓ AUC (32%), ↓ Cmax (37%) – unboosted	FDA document

AUC area-under-the curve, *Cmax* maximum concentration

significantly increased the AUC (18%) and Cmax (15%) of unboosted amprenavir under steady-state conditions, an effect likely explained by the inhibitory effects of clarithromycin toward CYP3A4 [69]. Both ketoconazole (200 mg daily, $N = 15$) and posaconazole (400 mg daily, $N=24$) had little effects on the pharmacokinetics of boosted-amprenavir (700 mg boosted by 100 mg ritonavir twice daily), whereas ketoconazole (400 mg as a single dose, $N=12$) was able to increase the exposure (31%) of unboosted amprenavir (1200 mg as a single dose). The discrepancy between boosted and unboosted amprenavir is clearly apparent, because contrary to expectations, potent inhibitors of CYP3A4 such as ketoconazole and posaconazole had little effects on the pharmacokinetics of amprenavir. These contradictory findings are consistent with the likelihood that the mixed enzyme induction/inhibition effects of the pharmacological booster ritonavir may have confounded the observation. On the other hand, the effects of ketoconazole on unboosted amprenavir can likely be explained by CYP3A4 inhibition.

Differences in the pharmacokinetic interaction between boosted versus unboosted amprenavir can also be demonstrated with rifabutin and rifampin [65]. Rifabutin (300 mg as a single dose, $N=30$) significantly increased the AUC (35 %) and Cmax (36 %) of steady-state boosted amprenavir (700 mg twice daily boosted with 100 mg ritonavir), when compared to the historical control. In contrast, both steady-state rifabutin (300 mg daily, $N=5$) and rifampin (300 mg daily, $N=11$) reduced the exposure of unboosted amprenavir (1200 mg twice daily). The discrepancy between boosted and unboosted amprenavir is clearly apparent, because contrary to expectations, rifabutin (a potent CYP3A4 inducer) uncharacteristically increased the exposure of boosted amprenavir, a finding that may be explained by the confounding enzyme induction/inhibition effects of the pharmacological booster ritonavir. On the other hand, the effects of rifabutin and rifampin on unboosted amprenavir can likely be explained by CYP3A4 induction; and, as further support of the mechanism of the interaction, the extent of changes in amprenavir exposure corresponded with the potency of the inducing agent (i.e., rifampin > rifabutin).

5.3.3.3   Miscellaneous Agents

The effects of atorvastatin (10 mg daily, $N=16$), esomeprazole (20 mg daily, $N=25$), ethinyl estradiol/norethindrone (0.035 mg/0.5 mg daily), methadone (70–120 mg daily, $N=19$), and phenytoin (300 mg daily, $N=13$) on the pharmacokinetics of amprenavir (± ritonavir) have been determined [65]. Atorvastatin decreased the AUC (27 %) of boosted amprenavir (700 mg twice daily with 100 mg ritonavir) but had little effect toward the exposure of unboosted amprenavir (1400 mg twice daily) under steady-state conditions. The effects of atorvastatin (substrate and weak inhibitor of CYP3A4) [70] on boosted amprenavir might be confounded by the concurrent enzyme inducing effects of the co-administered ritonavir. On the other hand, the apparent lack of effects of atorvastatin on unboosted amprenavir suggests little inhibition potential from atorvastatin toward CYP3A4, although this assertion remains to be tested. Because amprenavir is capable of increasing the exposure of atorvastatin (Chap. 6), the co-administration of these drugs would not be recommended.

Esomeprazole and ethinyl estradiol/norethindrone did not affect the pharmacokinetics of amprenavir (± ritonavir). This finding is expected because there is very little pharmacological basis for esomeprazole or ethinyl-estradiol to modulate CYP3A4. On the other hand, methadone had little effects on the exposure of boosted amprenavir (700 mg twice daily with 100 mg ritonavir), but significantly decreased the AUC (30 %) and Cmax (27 %) of unboosted amprenavir (1200 mg twice daily) under steady-state conditions. It is unclear why methadone (not known to induce CYP3A4) would reduce the exposure of unboosted amprenavir and why this effect would be diminished in the presence of ritonavir. Perhaps the lack of adequate controls in these experiments (comparison was to historical control only) may have yielded unintended confounders. Likewise, the effects of phenytoin (a known

CYP3A4 inducer) on increased exposure of boosted amprenavir (700 mg twice daily with 100 mg ritonavir) do not correlate to the known pharmacological characteristics of either drug and might be confounded by the concurrent enzyme induction effects of the co-administered ritonavir.

5.3.4 *Indinavir* [71]/*Nelfinavir* [72]/*Lopinavir* [73–75]/ *Saquinavir* [76]/*Ritonavir* [77]/*Tipranavir* [78] (Tables 5.16, 5.17, 5.18, 5.19, and 5.20)

Indinavir, nelfinavir, lopinavir, saquinavir, and tipranavir (± ritonavir) have similar pharmacological characteristics compared to atazanavir, amprenavir, and darunavir (i.e., primarily a substrate and inhibitor of CYP3A4 and mixed pharmacological

Table 5.16 Effects of co-administered drugs on the pharmacokinetics of indinavir [71]

Drug	Summary effects on pharmacokinetics	Reference
Cimetidine	No significant change in pharmacokinetic parameters	FDA document
Clarithromycin	No significant change in pharmacokinetic parameters	FDA document
Fluconazole	↓ AUC (24%), ↓ Cmax (13%)	FDA document
Isoniazid	No significant change in pharmacokinetic parameters	FDA document
Itraconazole	No significant change in pharmacokinetic parameters	FDA document
Quinidine	No significant change in pharmacokinetic parameters	FDA document
Rifabutin	↓ AUC (32%), ↓ Cmax (20%)	FDA document
Rifampin	↓ AUC (92%), ↓ Cmax (87%)	FDA document

AUC area-under-the curve, *Cmax* maximum concentration

Table 5.17 Effects of co-administered drugs on the pharmacokinetics of nelfinavir [72]

Drug	Summary effects on pharmacokinetics	Reference
Azithromycin	↓ AUC (15%), ↓ Cmax (10%)	FDA document
Indinavir	↑ AUC (83%), ↑ Cmax (31%)	FDA document
Ketoconazole	↑ AUC (35%), ↑ Cmax (25%)	FDA document
Omeprazole	↓ AUC (36%), ↓ Cmax (37%)	FDA document
Phenytoin	No significant change in pharmacokinetic parameters	FDA document
Rifabutin	↓ AUC (23%), ↓ Cmax (18%)	FDA document
Rifampin	↓ AUC (83%), ↓ Cmax (76%)	FDA document
Ritonavir	↑ AUC (152%),↑ Cmax (44%)	FDA document
Saquinavir	↑ AUC (18%)	FDA document

AUC area-under-the curve, *Cmax* maximum concentration

Table 5.18 Effects of co-administered drugs on the pharmacokinetics of lopinavir (± ritonavir) [73–75]

Drug	Summary effects on pharmacokinetics	Reference
Boceprevir	↓ AUC (34 %), ↓ Cmax (30 %)	FDA document
Fosamprenavir	↑ AUC (37 %), ↑ Cmax (30 %)	FDA document
Lamotrigine	No significant changes in pharmacokinetic parameters	van der Lee 2006
Ketoconazole	↓ AUC (13 %), ↓ Cmax (11 %)	FDA document
Omeprazole	No significant changes in pharmacokinetic parameters	FDA document
Phenytoin	↓ AUC (31 %)	Lim 2004
Pravastatin	No significant changes in pharmacokinetic parameters	FDA document
Rifabutin	↑ AUC (17 %)	FDA document
Rifampin	↓ AUC (up to 75 % – depending on regimen of lopinavir/ ritonavir)	FDA document
Telaprevir	No significant changes in pharmacokinetic parameters	FDA document

AUC area-under-the curve, *Cmax* maximum concentration

Table 5.19 Effects of co-administered drugs on the pharmacokinetics of saquinavir (± ritonavir) [76]

Drug	Summary effects on pharmacokinetics	Reference
Atazanavir	↑ AUC (60 %), ↑ Cmax (42 %)	FDA document
Clarithromycin	↑ AUC (177 %), ↑ Cmax (187 %) – unboosted	FDA document
Indinavir	↑ AUC (364 %), ↑ Cmax (299 %) – unboosted	FDA document
Fosamprenavir	No significant effects in pharmacokinetic parameters	FDA document
Ketoconazole	No significant effects in pharmacokinetic parameters	FDA document
Omeprazole	↑ AUC (82 %), ↑ Cmax (75 %)	FDA document
Rifabutin	↓ AUC (47 %), ↓ Cmax (39 %)	FDA document
Ritonavir	↑ AUC (121 %), ↑ Cmax (64 %)	FDA document

AUC area-under-the curve, *Cmax* maximum concentration

Table 5.20 Effects of co-administered drugs on the pharmacokinetics of tipranavir (± ritonavir) [78]

Drug	Summary effects on pharmacokinetics	Reference
Atazanavir/ ritonavir	↑ AUC (20 %)	FDA document
Clarithromycin	↑ AUC (66 %), ↑ Cmax (40 %)	FDA document
Ethinyl estradiol/ norethindrone	No significant changes in pharmacokinetic parameters	FDA document
Fluconazole	↑ AUC (50 %), ↑ Cmax (32 %)	FDA document
Loperamide	No significant changes in pharmacokinetic parameters	FDA document
Rifabutin	No significant changes in pharmacokinetic parameters	FDA document
Rosuvastatin	No significant changes in pharmacokinetic parameters	FDA document
Tadalafil	No significant changes in pharmacokinetic parameters	FDA document

AUC area-under-the curve, *Cmax* maximum concentration

effects with the boosting agent ritonavir); thus, they would exhibit comparable pharmacokinetic interactions as discussed for these protease inhibitors, with slight variations. See Tables 5.16, 5.17, 5.18, 5.19, and 5.20 for the summaries of pharmacokinetic interactions observed with these agents. Because ritonavir is never administered alone, its interaction effects (when combined as a boosting pharmacological agent) are presented with the other antiviral agents.

5.4   Fusion Inhibitors

5.4.1   *Enfuvirtide* (Table 5.21)

Few drug-drug interactions are expected to be associated with enfuvirtide because it is not known to be extensively metabolized by the common Phase I (CYP450) or Phase II (UGT) enzymes or transported by Phase III transporters (Chap. 4). The effects of ritonavir, saquinavir/ritonavir, and rifampin on the pharmacokinetics of enfuvirtide have been characterized by the manufacturer [79], but, to our knowledge, no other information has been reported in the literature. In HIV-positive patients, ritonavir (200 mg every 12 h for 4 days, $N = 12$) significantly increased the AUC (22 %) and Cmax (24 %) of enfuvirtide (90 mg twice daily), whereas saquinavir/ritonavir (1000 mg/100 mg, every 12 h for 4 days, $N = 12$) and rifampin (600 mg once daily for 10 days, $N = 12$) did not have significant effects. More importantly, these effects were not related to significant changes in pharmacodynamic actions of enfuvirtide; thus, the documented pharmacokinetic change with ritonavir would not be clinically relevant. The effects of ritonavir on enfuvirtide exposure is unlikely mediated by metabolism-based inactivation, based on the known metabolism characteristics of these drugs. As such, other pharmacokinetic processes such as absorption or excretion might be involved, but further experiments in human are needed to verify this hypothesis. The lack of effects of saquinavir/ritonavir (mixed inhibitor/inducer) and rifampin (potent CYP3A4 inducer) on the pharmacokinetics of enfuvirtide confirms the general lack of metabolism-mediated interaction associated with enfuvirtide.

Table 5.21 Effects of co-administered drugs on the pharmacokinetics of enfuvirtide [79]

Drug	Summary effects on pharmacokinetics	Reference
Ritonavir	↑ AUC (22 %), ↑ Cmax (24 %)	FDA document
Saquinavir/ritonavir	No significant effects on pharmacokinetic parameters	FDA document
Rifampin	No significant effects on pharmacokinetic parameters	FDA document

AUC area-under-the curve, *Cmax* maximum concentration

5.5 Entry Inhibitors

5.5.1 *Maraviroc* (Table 5.22)

The effects of protease inhibitors (atazanavir/ritonavir, fosamprenavir/ritonavir, lopinavir/ritonavir, ritonavir, saquinavir/ritonavir, and tipranavir/ritonavir) on the pharmacokinetics of maraviroc have been characterized in humans [80, 81]. Atazanavir/ritonavir (300 mg/100 mg daily), fosamprenavir/ritonavir (700 mg/100 mg twice daily), lopinavir/ritonavir (400 mg/100 mg twice daily), ritonavir (100 mg twice daily), and saquinavir/ritonavir (1000 mg/100 mg twice daily) all increased the AUC (388%, 149%, 295%, 161%, 877%, respectively) of maraviroc (100–300 mg twice daily, $N = 8\text{-}12$) under steady-state conditions, but tipranavir/ritonavir (500 mg/200 mg twice daily) had little effects. These significant interactions (except for tipranavir) are likely mediated by the protease inhibitors' inhibitory effects toward CYP3A4, the primary enzyme responsible for the metabolism of maraviroc in humans [82]. The lack of significant interaction between tipranavir/ritonavir and maraviroc might be secondary to the mixed inhibition/induction effects of tipranavir or ritonavir toward CYP450 and transporters that mediate the clearance of maraviroc. Overall, these data indicate that significant dose adjustment is needed when maraviroc is co-administered with protease inhibitors.

Consistent with the findings obtained with protease inhibitors, the co-administration of maraviroc with other CYP3A4 inhibitors such as boceprevir, ketoconazole (but not nevirapine) or CYP3A4 inducers such as efavirenz and rifampin has also produced significant pharmacokinetic interactions [80, 83]. Boceprevir (300 mg three times daily) and ketoconazole (400 mg daily) both significantly

Table 5.22 Effects of co-administered drugs on the pharmacokinetics of maraviroc [80–83]

Drug	Summary effects on pharmacokinetics	Reference
Atazanavir/ritonavir	↑ AUC (388%), ↑ Cmax (167%)	FDA document
Boceprevir	↑ AUC (142%)	Vourvahis 2014
Efavirenz	↓ AUC (45%), ↓ Cmax (52%)	FDA document
Fosamprenavir/ritonavir	↑ AUC (149%), ↑ Cmax (45%)	Vourvahis 2013
Ketoconazole	↑ AUC (400%), ↑ Cmax (238%)	FDA document
Lopinavir/ritonavir	↑ AUC (295%), ↑ Cmax (97%)	FDA document
Nevirapine	No significant changes in pharmacokinetic parameters	FDA document
Rifampin	↓ AUC (64%), ↓ Cmax (66%)	FDA document
Ritonavir	↑ AUC (161%), ↑ Cmax (28%)	FDA document
Saquinavir/ritonavir	↑ AUC (877%), ↑ Cmax (378%)	FDA document
Tipranavir/ritonavir	No significant changes in pharmacokinetic parameters	FDA document

AUC area-under-the curve, *Cmax* maximum concentration

increased the AUC of maraviroc by 142 % and 400 %, respectively, whereas nevirapine (200 mg twice daily, with lamivudine 150 mg twice daily and tenofovir 300 mg daily) had little effects on the exposure of maraviroc. The findings with boceprevir and ketoconazole are likely associated with the inhibition of CYP3A4, those of efavirenz and rifampin are explained by the induction of CYP3A4, and the lack of significant pharmacokinetic interaction with nevirapine is consistent with to the nonpotent inhibitory effects of the NNRTI toward the same enzyme [84]. Taken together, these data suggest that other CYP3A4 modulators would likely affect the pharmacokinetics of maraviroc in a predictable manner and that dose adjustment is needed when modulators of CYP3A4 are co-administered with maraviroc.

5.6   Integrase Inhibitors

5.6.1   *Dolutegravir* (Table 5.23)

5.6.1.1   Protease Inhibitors

The effects of various protease inhibitors (atazanavir, atazanavir/ritonavir, darunavir/ritonavir, fosamprenavir/ritonavir, lopinavir/ritonavir, and tipranavir/ritonavir) on the pharmacokinetics of dolutegravir have been determined in humans [85]. Atazanavir (400 mg daily, $n = 12$) or boosted atazanavir (300 mg with 100 mg ritonavir, $N = 12$) significantly increased the AUC (91 % and 62 %, respectively) and

Table 5.23 Effects of co-administered drugs on the pharmacokinetics of dolutegravir [85]

Drug	Summary effects on pharmacokinetics	Reference
Atazanavir	↑ AUC (91 %), ↑ Cmax (50 %)	FDA document
Atazanavir/ ritonavir	↑ AUC (62 %), ↑ Cmax (34 %)	FDA document
Boceprevir	No significant changes in pharmacokinetic parameters	FDA document
Darunavir/ritonavir	↓ AUC (22 %)	FDA document
Efavirenz	↓ AUC (57 %), ↓ Cmax (39 %)	FDA document
Fosamprenavir/ ritonavir	No significant changes in pharmacokinetic parameters	FDA document
Lopinavir/ritonavir	No significant changes in pharmacokinetic parameters	FDA document
Omeprazole	No significant changes in pharmacokinetic parameters	FDA document
Prednisone	↑ AUC (11 %)	FDA document
Rifabutin	No significant changes in pharmacokinetic parameters	FDA document
Rifampin	↓ AUC (54 %), ↓ Cmax (43 %)	FDA document
Tenofovir	No significant changes in pharmacokinetic parameters	FDA document
Rilpivirine	↑ AUC (12 %)	FDA document
Tipranavir/ ritonavir	↓ AUC (59 %), ↓ Cmax (46 %)	FDA document
Telaprevir	↑ AUC (25 %), ↑ Cmax (18 %)	FDA document

AUC area-under-the curve, *Cmax* maximum concentration

Cmax (50% and 34%, respectively) of dolutegravir (30 mg daily) under steady-state conditions. These effects are consistent with the known metabolic characteristics of dolutegravir (primarily metabolized by UGT1A1 and CYP3A4 enzymes) [86] and atazanavir (inhibitors of both UGT1A1 and CYP3A4) [57]. Atazanavir boosted by ritonavir had apparently reduced inhibitory effect toward dolutegravir metabolism, and this may be explained by the induction effects of ritonavir, which may have offset the inhibitory effects of atazanavir. These findings suggest that the co-administration of these agents is not recommended.

In contrast to atazanavir, darunavir (600 mg boosted by ritonavir 100 mg twice daily, $N = 15$), fosamprenavir (700 mg boosted by 100 mg ritonavir twice daily, $N = 12$), lopinavir (400 mg boosted by 100 mg ritonavir twice daily, $N = 15$), and tipranavir (750 mg boosted by 200 mg ritonavir twice daily, $N = 14$) had little effects on the pharmacokinetics (fosamprenavir, lopinavir) or decreased the exposure (darunavir, tipranavir) of dolutegravir. These findings are contradictory to the known inhibitory effects of these protease inhibitors toward CYP3A4 (Chap. 4), which in theory should increase (rather than decrease) the exposure of dolutegravir, a primary metabolite of the same enzyme [86]. However, these experiments were also potentially confounded by the induction effects of co-administered ritonavir and tipranavir itself toward UGT enzymes [87], which may be responsible for the conjugation of dolutegravir. Overall, mixed effects of protease inhibitors on the pharmacokinetics of dolutegravir have been documented, and clinicians should be aware of the inconsistent/opposite effects these agents may have on the pharmacokinetics of dolutegravir, which may require some dose adjustment.

5.6.1.2   Other Antivirals

The effects of antihepatitis C antivirals (boceprevir, telaprevir), NNRTIs (efavirenz, rilpivirine), and NRTI (tenofovir) on the pharmacokinetics of dolutegravir have been determined [85]. Boceprevir (800 mg every 8 h, $N = 13$) did not change the pharmacokinetics of dolutegravir, whereas telaprevir (750 mg every 8 h, $N = 15$) significantly increased the AUC (25%) and Cmax (18%) of dolutegravir (50 mg daily) under steady-state conditions. These effects are inconsistent (boceprevir) and supportive (telaprevir) of their known strong inhibitory effects toward CYP3A4 [30, 88], suggesting, in the case of boceprevir, other pharmacokinetic factors of dolutegravir may have been altered. However, the effects of telaprevir on the exposure of dolutegravir appear relatively minor and would likely not be clinically significant or warrant dose adjustment.

5.6.1.3   Other Drugs

The effects of omeprazole, prednisone, rifabutin, and rifampin on the pharmacokinetics of dolutegravir have been characterized [85]. Omeprazole (40 mg daily, $N = 12$), prednisone (60 mg daily, $N = 12$), and rifabutin (600 mg once daily, $N = 11$)

did not have significant effects on the pharmacokinetics of dolutegravir (50 mg single dose or twice daily), whereas rifampin (600 mg once daily, $N=11$) modestly increased the exposure (33 %) and Cmax (18 %) of dolutegravir (50 mg twice daily) in human subjects. The lack of effects of omeprazole and prednisone is consistent with the lack of pharmacological basis (i.e., no documented inhibitory or induction effects toward CYP3A4 and UGT1A1 known to mediate the metabolism of dolutegravir) by these agents to mediate metabolism-associated drug interaction with dolutegravir. On the other hand, despite being a known inducer of CYP3A4 and UGT enzymes, rifabutin had little effects on the exposure, but rifampin significantly increased the exposure (54 %) and Cmax (43 %) of dolutegravir, suggesting the use of rifabutin over rifampin if required. These findings also indicate that relatively potent inducers (i.e., rifampin) are more likely to cause a change in the pharmacokinetics of dolutegravir despite the lack of drug interaction potential of dolutegravir in general.

5.6.2   *Elvitegravir* [89] *and Raltegravir* [90] (Tables 5.24 and 5.25)

Elvitegravir and raltegravir exhibit similar metabolism characteristics compared to dolutegravir (Chap. 4) and thus have comparable, albeit slightly variable, clinical pharmacokinetic interactions. See Tables 5.24 and 5.25 for the documented pharmacokinetic interactions observed in humans.

Table 5.24 Effects of co-administered drugs on the pharmacokinetics of elvitegravir (± ritonavir) [89]

Drug	Summary effects on pharmacokinetics	Reference
Atazanavir	↑ AUC (100 %), ↑ Cmax (85 %)	FDA document
Darunavir	No significant changes in pharmacokinetic parameters	FDA document
Didanosine	No significant changes in pharmacokinetic parameters	FDA document
Ketoconazole	↑ AUC (48 %), ↑ Cmax (17 %)	FDA document
Lopinavir/ritonavir	↑ AUC (75 %), ↑ Cmax (52 %)	FDA document
Rifabutin	No significant changes in pharmacokinetic parameters	FDA document
Rosuvastatin	No significant changes in pharmacokinetic parameters	FDA document
Tipranavir	No significant changes in pharmacokinetic parameters	FDA document

AUC area-under-the curve, *Cmax* maximum concentration

Table 5.25   Effects of co-administered drugs on the pharmacokinetics of raltegravir [90]

Drug	Summary effects on pharmacokinetics	Reference
Atazanavir	↑ AUC (72%), ↑ Cmax (53%)	FDA document
Atazanavir/ritonavir	↑ AUC (41%), ↑ Cmax (24%)	FDA document
Efavirenz	↓ AUC (36%), ↓ Cmax (36%)	FDA document
Etravirine	No significant effects on pharmacokinetic parameters	FDA document
Methadone	No significant effects on pharmacokinetic parameters	FDA document
Rifampin	↓ AUC (40%), ↓ Cmax (38%)	FDA document
Ritonavir	No significant effects on pharmacokinetic parameters	FDA document
Tenofovir	↑ AUC (49%), ↑ Cmax (64%)	FDA document
Tipranavir/ritonavir	No significant effects on pharmacokinetic parameters	FDA document

AUC area-under-the curve, *Cmax* maximum concentration

5.7   Summary

Most of the effects of co-administered drugs on the pharmacokinetics of antiviral agents might be explained by the known metabolic characteristics already established from in vitro studies (Chap. 4). The NNRTIs, PIs, and the fusion inhibitor maraviroc are primarily metabolized by CYP450 enzymes (where CYP3A4 plays a major role) and are thus subject to interacting effects from known modulators of these systems. Moreover, due to mixed induction/inhibition characteristics exhibited by some NNRTIs and PIs, the simple paradigm of one-modulator, one-substrate interaction does not always hold true, as multiple enzymes and drugs are usually involved and the antiretroviral drugs may also exhibit mixed inhibition/induction properties themselves. On the other hand, the NRTIs and the fusion inhibitor enfuvirtide are not subject to drug interactions mediated by CYP or UGT enzymes, and clinical data confirm few metabolism-mediated reactions with these substrates. The exception within the NRTI class is zidovudine, which exhibits similar metabolic characteristics as the integrase inhibitors (dolutegravir, elvitegravir, and raltegravir) and is subject to interacting effects from UGT inhibitors or inducers.

The common limitations observed in the reported clinical pharmacokinetic studies are (i) small sample sizes, (ii) lack of reporting of additional pharmacokinetic data other than drug exposure and concentrations (which limits the mechanistic interpretation of the reported interaction), and (iii) lack of correlation with pharmacodynamic effects. In general, future studies should ideally focus on collecting the full spectrum of pharmacokinetic data within the HIV-positive patient population and draw correlations to the pharmacodynamic effects already reported in the literature.

References

1. Guidelines for the use of antiretroviral agents in HIV-1-infected adults and adolescents. 2016; Available at: https://aidsinfo.nih.gov/guidelines/html/1/adult-and-adolescent-treatment-guidelines/0. Accessed 19 June 2016
2. McCance-Katz EF, Moody DE, Morse GD, Friedland G, Pade P, Baker J et al (2006) Interactions between buprenorphine and antiretrovirals. I. The nonnucleoside reverse-transcriptase inhibitors efavirenz and delavirdine. Clin Infect Dis 43(Suppl 4):S224–S234
3. Voorman RL, Maio SM, Payne NA, Zhao Z, Koeplinger KA, Wang X (1998) Microsomal metabolism of delavirdine: evidence for mechanism-based inactivation of human cytochrome P450 3A. J Pharmacol Exp Ther 287(1):381–388
4. Kobayashi K, Yamamoto T, Chiba K, Tani M, Shimada N, Ishizaki T et al (1998) Human buprenorphine N-dealkylation is catalyzed by cytochrome P450 3A4. Drug Metab Dispos 26(8):818–821
5. Rescriptor (2012) Prescribing information. Available at: http://www.accessdata.fda.gov/drugsatfda_docs/label/2012/020705s018lbl.pdf. Accessed 19 June 2016
6. Ito K, Ogihara K, Kanamitsu S, Itoh T (2003) Prediction of the in vivo interaction between midazolam and macrolides based on in vitro studies using human liver microsomes. Drug Metab Dispos 31(7):945–954
7. Borin MT, Cox SR, Herman BD, Carel BJ, Anderson RD, Freimuth WW (1997) Effect of fluconazole on the steady-state pharmacokinetics of delavirdine in human immunodeficiency virus-positive patients. Antimicrob Agents Chemother 41(9):1892–1897
8. Niwa T, Shiraga T, Takagi A (2005) Effect of antifungal drugs on cytochrome P450 (CYP) 2C9, CYP2C19, and CYP3A4 activities in human liver microsomes. Biol Pharm Bull 28(9):1805–1808
9. Borin MT, Chambers JH, Carel BJ, Gagnon S, Freimuth WW (1997) Pharmacokinetic study of the interaction between rifampin and delavirdine mesylate. Clin Pharmacol Ther 61(5):544–553
10. Borin MT, Chambers JH, Carel BJ, Freimuth WW, Aksentijevich S, Piergies AA (1997) Pharmacokinetic study of the interaction between rifabutin and delavirdine mesylate in HIV-1 infected patients. Antiviral Res 35(1):53–63
11. Ferry JJ, Herman BD, Carel BJ, Carlson GF, Batts DH (1998) Pharmacokinetic drug-drug interaction study of delavirdine and indinavir in healthy volunteers. J Acquir Immune Defic Syndr Hum Retrovirol 18(3):252–259
12. Morse GD, Fischl MA, Shelton MJ, Cox SR, Driver M, DeRemer M et al (1997) Single-dose pharmacokinetics of delavirdine mesylate and didanosine in patients with human immunodeficiency virus infection. Antimicrob Agents Chemother 41(1):169–174
13. Sustiva (2008) Prescribing information. Available at: http://www.accessdata.fda.gov/drugsatfda_docs/label/2008/020972s030,021360s019lbl.pdf. Accessed 19 June 2016
14. Burt HJ, Galetin A, Houston JB (2010) IC50-based approaches as an alternative method for assessment of time-dependent inhibition of CYP3A4. Xenobiotica 40(5):331–343
15. Williamson B, Dooley KE, Zhang Y, Back DJ, Owen A (2013) Induction of influx and efflux transporters and cytochrome P450 3A4 in primary human hepatocytes by rifampin, rifabutin, and rifapentine. Antimicrob Agents Chemother 57(12):6366–6369
16. Ji P, Damle B, Xie J, Unger SE, Grasela DM, Kaul S (2008) Pharmacokinetic interaction between efavirenz and carbamazepine after multiple-dose administration in healthy subjects. J Clin Pharmacol 48(8):948–956
17. Sekar VJ, De Pauw M, Marien K, Peeters M, Lefebvre E, Hoetelmans RM (2007) Pharmacokinetic interaction between TMC114/r and efavirenz in healthy volunteers. Antivir Ther 12(4):509–514
18. Arya V (2005) Clinical pharmacology and biopharmaceutics review (21–976). Available at: http://www.accessdata.fda.gov/drugsatfda_docs/nda/2006/021976s000_Sprycel_ClinPharmR.pdf. Accessed 6 June 2016

19. Kumar GN, Rodrigues AD, Buko AM, Denissen JF (1996) Cytochrome P450-mediated metabolism of the HIV-1 protease inhibitor ritonavir (ABT-538) in human liver microsomes. J Pharmacol Exp Ther 277(1):423–431

20. Eagling VA, Back DJ, Barry MG (1997) Differential inhibition of cytochrome P450 isoforms by the protease inhibitors, ritonavir, saquinavir and indinavir. Br J Clin Pharmacol 44(2):190–194

21. Lillibridge JH, Liang BH, Kerr BM, Webber S, Quart B, Shetty BV et al (1998) Characterization of the selectivity and mechanism of human cytochrome P450 inhibition by the human immunodeficiency virus-protease inhibitor nelfinavir mesylate. Drug Metab Dispos 26(7):609–616

22. Granfors MT, Wang JS, Kajosaari LI, Laitila J, Neuvonen PJ, Backman JT (2006) Differential inhibition of cytochrome P450 3A4, 3A5 and 3A7 by five human immunodeficiency virus (HIV) protease inhibitors in vitro. Basic Clin Pharmacol Toxicol 98(1):79–85

23. Liu L, Mugundu GM, Kirby BJ, Samineni D, Desai PB, Unadkat JD (2012) Quantification of human hepatocyte cytochrome P450 enzymes and transporters induced by HIV protease inhibitors using newly validated LC-MS/MS cocktail assays and RT-PCR. Biopharm Drug Dispos 33(4):207–217

24. Kakuda TN, DeMasi R, van Delft Y, Mohammed P (2013) Pharmacokinetic interaction between etravirine or darunavir/ritonavir and artemether/lumefantrine in healthy volunteers: a two-panel, two-way, two-period, randomized trial. HIV Med 14(7):421–429

25. Intelence (2009) Prescribing information. Available at: http://www.accessdata.fda.gov/drugsatfda_docs/label/2009/022187s002lbl.pdf. Accessed 19 June 2016

26. Kakuda TN, Van Solingen-Ristea R, Aharchi F, Smedt GD, Witek J, Nijs S et al (2013) Pharmacokinetics and short-term safety of etravirine in combination with fluconazole or voriconazole in HIV-negative volunteers. J Clin Pharmacol 53(1):41–50

27. Yanakakis LJ, Bumpus NN (2012) Biotransformation of the antiretroviral drug etravirine: metabolite identification, reaction phenotyping, and characterization of autoinduction of cytochrome P450-dependent metabolism. Drug Metab Dispos 40(4):803–814

28. Hammond KP, Wolfe P, Burton JR Jr, Predhomme JA, Ellis CM, Ray ML et al (2013) Pharmacokinetic interaction between boceprevir and etravirine in HIV/HCV seronegative volunteers. J Acquir Immune Defic Syndr 62(1):67–73

29. Ogilvie BW, Yerino P, Kazmi F, Buckley DB, Rostami-Hodjegan A, Paris BL et al (2011) The proton pump inhibitor, omeprazole, but not lansoprazole or pantoprazole, is a metabolism-dependent inhibitor of CYP2C19: implications for coadministration with clopidogrel. Drug Metab Dispos 39(11):2020–2033

30. Chu X, Cai X, Cui D, Tang C, Ghosal A, Chan G et al (2013) In vitro assessment of drug-drug interaction potential of boceprevir associated with drug metabolizing enzymes and transporters. Drug Metab Dispos 41(3):668–681

31. Ernest CS 2nd, Hall SD, Jones DR (2005) Mechanism-based inactivation of CYP3A by HIV protease inhibitors. J Pharmacol Exp Ther 312(2):583–591

32. Viramune (2010) Prescribing information. Available at: http://www.accessdata.fda.gov/drugsatfda_docs/label/2010/020933s022,020636s032lbl.pdf. Accessed 19 June 2016

33. Edurant (2015) Prescribing information. Available at: http://www.edurant.com/shared/product/Edurant/EDURANT-PI.pdf. Accessed 19 June 2016

34. Lade JM, Avery LB, Bumpus NN (2013) Human biotransformation of the nonnucleoside reverse transcriptase inhibitor rilpivirine and a cross-species metabolism comparison. Antimicrob Agents Chemother 57(10):5067–5079

35. McDowell JA, Chittick GE, Ravitch JR, Polk RE, Kerkering TM, Stein DS (1999) Pharmacokinetics of [(14)C]abacavir, a human immunodeficiency virus type 1 (HIV-1) reverse transcriptase inhibitor, administered in a single oral dose to HIV-1-infected adults: a mass balance study. Antimicrob Agents Chemother 43(12):2855–2861

36. Boelaert JR, Dom GM, Huitema AD, Beijnen JH, Lange JM (2002) The boosting of didanosine by allopurinol permits a halving of the didanosine dosage. AIDS 16(16):2221–2223

37. Videx (2009) Prescribing information. Available at: http://www.accessdata.fda.gov/drug-satfda_docs/label/2009/020156s044lbl.pdf. Accessed 19 June 2016

38. Ray AS, Olson L, Fridland A (2004) Role of purine nucleoside phosphorylase in interactions between 2′,3′-dideoxyinosine and allopurinol, ganciclovir, or tenofovir. Antimicrob Agents Chemother 48(4):1089–1095

39. Emtriva (2012) Prescribing information. Available at: http://www.gilead.com/~/media/files/pdfs/medicines/hiv/emtriva/emtriva_pi.pdf. Accessed 19 June 2016

40. Epivir (2013) Prescribing information. Available at: https://www.viivhealthcare.com/media/32160/us_epivir.pdf. Accessed 19 June 2016

41. Zerit (2008) Prescribing information. Available at: http://www.accessdata.fda.gov/drugsatfda_docs/label/2008/020412s029,020413s020lbl.pdf. Accessed 19 June 2016

42. Rainey PM, Friedland G, McCance-Katz EF, Andrews L, Mitchell SM, Charles C et al (2000) Interaction of methadone with didanosine and stavudine. J Acquir Immune Defic Syndr 24(3):241–248

43. Viread (2012) Prescribing information. Available at: http://www.accessdata.fda.gov/drug-satfda_docs/label/2012/021356s042,022577s002lbl.pdf. Accessed 19 June 2016

44. Baker J, Rainey PM, Moody DE, Morse GD, Ma Q, McCance-Katz EF (2010) Interactions between buprenorphine and antiretrovirals: nucleos(t)ide reverse transcriptase inhibitors (NRTI) didanosine, lamivudine, and tenofovir. Am J Addict 19(1):17–29

45. Wenning LA, Friedman EJ, Kost JT, Breidinger SA, Stek JE, Lasseter KC et al (2008) Lack of a significant drug interaction between raltegravir and tenofovir. Antimicrob Agents Chemother 52(9):3253–3258

46. Barbier O, Turgeon D, Girard C, Green MD, Tephly TR, Hum DW et al (2000) 3′-azido-3′-deoxythimidine (AZT) is glucuronidated by human UDP-glucuronosyltransferase 2B7 (UGT2B7). Drug Metab Dispos 28(5):497–502

47. Trapnell CB, Klecker RW, Jamis-Dow C, Collins JM (1998) Glucuronidation of 3′-azido-3′-deoxythymidine (zidovudine) by human liver microsomes: relevance to clinical pharmacokinetic interactions with atovaquone, fluconazole, methadone, and valproic acid. Antimicrob Agents Chemother 42(7):1592–1596

48. Belanger AS, Caron P, Harvey M, Zimmerman PA, Mehlotra RK, Guillemette C (2009) Glucuronidation of the antiretroviral drug efavirenz by UGT2B7 and an in vitro investigation of drug-drug interaction with zidovudine. Drug Metab Dispos 37(9):1793–1796

49. Uchaipichat V, Winner LK, Mackenzie PI, Elliot DJ, Williams JA, Miners JO (2006) Quantitative prediction of in vivo inhibitory interactions involving glucuronidated drugs from in vitro data: the effect of fluconazole on zidovudine glucuronidation. Br J Clin Pharmacol 61(4):427–439

50. Raungrut P, Uchaipichat V, Elliot DJ, Janchawee B, Somogyi AA, Miners JO (2010) In vitro-in vivo extrapolation predicts drug-drug interactions arising from inhibition of codeine glucuronidation by dextropropoxyphene, fluconazole, ketoconazole, and methadone in humans. J Pharmacol Exp Ther 334(2):609–618

51. Uchaipichat V, Mackenzie PI, Guo XH, Gardner-Stephen D, Galetin A, Houston JB et al (2004) Human udp-glucuronosyltransferases: isoform selectivity and kinetics of 4-methylumbelliferone and 1-naphthol glucuronidation, effects of organic solvents, and inhibition by diclofenac and probenecid. Drug Metab Dispos 32(4):413–423

52. Ethell BT, Anderson GD, Burchell B (2003) The effect of valproic acid on drug and steroid glucuronidation by expressed human UDP-glucuronosyltransferases. Biochem Pharmacol 65(9):1441–1449

53. Retrovir (2008) Prescribing information. Available at: http://www.accessdata.fda.gov/drug-satfda_docs/label/2008/019910s033lbl.pdf. Accessed 19 June 2016

54. Gallicano KD, Sahai J, Shukla VK, Seguin I, Pakuts A, Kwok D et al (1999) Induction of zidovudine glucuronidation and amination pathways by rifampicin in HIV-infected patients. Br J Clin Pharmacol 48(2):168–179

55. Ouellet D, Hsu A, Qian J, Locke CS, Eason CJ, Cavanaugh JH et al (1998) Effect of ritonavir on the pharmacokinetics of ethinyl oestradiol in healthy female volunteers. Br J Clin Pharmacol 46(2):111–116

56. Hulskotte EG, Feng HP, Xuan F, van Zutven MG, Treitel MA, Hughes EA et al (2013) Pharmacokinetic interactions between the hepatitis C virus protease inhibitor boceprevir and ritonavir-boosted HIV-1 protease inhibitors atazanavir, darunavir, and lopinavir. Clin Infect Dis 56(5):718–726

57. Zheng J (2002) Clinical pharmacology and biopharmaceutics review (21–567). Available at: http://www.accessdata.fda.gov/drugsatfda_docs/nda/2003/21-567_Reyataz_BioPharmr_P1.pdf. Accessed 6 June 2016

58. Reyataz (2015) Prescribing information. Available at: http://packageinserts.bms.com/pi/pi_reyataz.pdf. Accessed 19 June 2016

59. Zhang X, Jones DR, Hall SD (2009) Prediction of the effect of erythromycin, diltiazem, and their metabolites, alone and in combination, on CYP3A4 inhibition. Drug Metab Dispos 37(1):150–160

60. Krishna G, Moton A, Ma L, Martinho M, Seiberling M, McLeod J (2009) Effects of oral posaconazole on the pharmacokinetics of atazanavir alone and with ritonavir or with efavirenz in healthy adult volunteers. J Acquir Immune Defic Syndr 51(4):437–444

61. Michaud V, Turgeon J (2010) Assessment of competitive and mechanism-based inhibition by clarithromycin: use of domperidone as a CYP3A probe-drug substrate and various enzymatic sources including a new cell-based assay with freshly isolated human hepatocytes. Drug Metab Lett 4(2):69–76

62. Prezista (2015) Prescribing information. Available at: https://www.prezista.com/sites/default/files/pdf/us_package_insert.pdf. Accessed 19 June 2016

63. Chapron B, Risler L, Phillips B, Collins C, Thummel K, Shen D (2015) Reversible, time-dependent inhibition of CYP3A-mediated metabolism of midazolam and tacrolimus by tela-previr in human liver microsomes. J Pharm Pharm Sci 18(1):101–111

64. Magnusson MO, Dahl ML, Cederberg J, Karlsson MO, Sandstrom R (2008) Pharmacodynamics of carbamazepine-mediated induction of CYP3A4, CYP1A2, and Pgp as assessed by probe substrates midazolam, caffeine, and digoxin. Clin Pharmacol Ther 84(1):52–62

65. Lexiva (2009) Prescribing information. Available at: https://www.accessdata.fda.gov/drugsatfda_docs/label/2009/021548s021,022116s005lbl.pdf. Accessed 19 June 2016

66. Decker CJ, Laitinen LM, Bridson GW, Raybuck SA, Tung RD, Chaturvedi PR (1998) Metabolism of amprenavir in liver microsomes: role of CYP3A4 inhibition for drug interactions. J Pharm Sci 87(7):803–807

67. Iribarne C, Berthou F, Carlhant D, Dreano Y, Picart D, Lohezic F et al (1998) Inhibition of methadone and buprenorphine N-dealkylations by three HIV-1 protease inhibitors. Drug Metab Dispos 26(3):257–260

68. Bruggemann RJ, van Luin M, Colbers EP, van den Dungen MW, Pharo C, Schouwenberg BJ et al (2010) Effect of posaconazole on the pharmacokinetics of fosamprenavir and vice versa in healthy volunteers. J Antimicrob Chemother 65(10):2188–2194

69. Rodrigues AD, Roberts EM, Mulford DJ, Yao Y, Ouellet D (1997) Oxidative metabolism of clarithromycin in the presence of human liver microsomes. Major role for the cytochrome P4503A (CYP3A) subfamily. Drug Metab Dispos 25(5):623–630

70. Park JE, Kim KB, Bae SK, Moon BS, Liu KH, Shin JG (2008) Contribution of cytochrome P450 3A4 and 3A5 to the metabolism of atorvastatin. Xenobiotica 38(9):1240–1251

71. Crixivan (2008) Prescribing information. Available at: http://www.accessdata.fda.gov/drugsatfda_docs/label/2008/020685s066lbl.pdf. Accessed 19 June 2016

72. Viracept (2011) Prescribing information. Available at: http://www.accessdata.fda.gov/drugsatfda_docs/label/2011/020778s035,020779s056,021503s017lbl.pdf. Accessed 19 June 2016

73. Kaletra (2013) Prescribing information. Available at: http://www.accessdata.fda.gov/drugsatfda_docs/label/2013/021226s037lbl.pdf. Accessed 19 June 2016

74. van der Lee MJ, Dawood L, ter Hofstede HJ, de Graaff-Teulen MJ, van Ewijk-Beneken Kolmer EW, Caliskan-Yassen N et al (2006) Lopinavir/ritonavir reduces lamotrigine plasma concentrations in healthy subjects. Clin Pharmacol Ther 80(2):159–168

75. Lim ML, Min SS, Eron JJ, Bertz RJ, Robinson M, Gaedigk A et al (2004) Coadministration of lopinavir/ritonavir and phenytoin results in two-way drug interaction through cytochrome P-450 induction. J Acquir Immune Defic Syndr 36(5):1034–1040

76. Invirase (2010) Prescribing information. Available at: http://www.accessdata.fda.gov/drug-satfda_docs/label/2010/020628s032,021785s009lbl.pdf. Accessed 19 June 2016
77. Norvir (2005) Prescribing information. Available at: http://www.accessdata.fda.gov/drug-satfda_docs/label/2005/020659s034,020945s017lbl.pdf. Accessed 19 June 2016
78. Aptivus (2009) Prescribing information. Available at: http://www.accessdata.fda.gov/drug-satfda_docs/label/2009/021814s006,022292s001lbl.pdf. Accessed 19 June 2016
79. Fuzeon (2011) Prescribing information. Available at: http://hivdb.stanford.edu/pages/linksPages/ENF_PI.pdf. Accessed 19 June 2016
80. Selzentry (2007) Prescribing information. Available at: http://www.accessdata.fda.gov/drug-satfda_docs/label/2007/022128lbl.pdf. Accessed 19 June 2016
81. Vourvahis M, Plotka A (2013) Mendes da Costa L, Fang A, Heera J. Pharmacokinetic interaction between maraviroc and fosamprenavir-ritonavir: an open-label, fixed-sequence study in healthy subjects. Antimicrob Agents Chemother 57(12):6158–6164
82. Hyland R, Dickins M, Collins C, Jones H, Jones B (2008) Maraviroc: in vitro assessment of drug-drug interaction potential. Br J Clin Pharmacol 66(4):498–507
83. Vourvahis M, Plotka A, Kantaridis C, Fang A, Heera J (2014) The effects of boceprevir and telaprevir on the pharmacokinetics of maraviroc: an open-label, fixed-sequence study in healthy volunteers. J Acquir Immune Defic Syndr 65(5):564–570
84. Erickson DA, Mather G, Trager WF, Levy RH, Keirns JJ (1999) Characterization of the in vitro biotransformation of the HIV-1 reverse transcriptase inhibitor nevirapine by human hepatic cytochromes P-450. Drug Metab Dispos 27(12):1488–1495
85. Tivicay (2013) Prescribing information. Available at: http://www.accessdata.fda.gov/drug-satfda_docs/label/2013/204790lbl.pdf. Accessed 19 June 2016
86. Reese MJ, Savina PM, Generaux GT, Tracey H, Humphreys JE, Kanaoka E et al (2013) In vitro investigations into the roles of drug transporters and metabolizing enzymes in the disposition and drug interactions of dolutegravir, a HIV integrase inhibitor. Drug Metab Dispos 41(2):353–361
87. Bruce RD, Moody DE, Fang WB, Chodkowski D, Andrews L, Friedland GH (2011) Tipranavir/ritonavir induction of buprenorphine glucuronide metabolism in HIV-negative subjects chronically receiving buprenorphine/naloxone. Am J Drug Alcohol Abuse 37(4):224–228
88. Kiang TK, Wilby KJ, Ensom MH (2013) Telaprevir: clinical pharmacokinetics, pharmacodynamics, and drug-drug interactions. Clin Pharmacokinet 52(7):487–510
89. Vitekta (2014) Prescribing information. Available at: https://www.accessdata.fda.gov/drug-satfda_docs/label/2014/203093s000lbl.pdf. Accessed 19 June 2016
90. Isentress (2011) Prescribing information. Available at: http://www.accessdata.fda.gov/drug-satfda_docs/label/2011/022145s018lbl.pdf. Accessed 19 June 2016

Chapter 6
Clinical Drug-Drug Interaction Data: Effects of Antiretroviral Agents on Co-administered Drugs

Tony K.L. Kiang, Kyle John Wilby, and Mary H.H. Ensom

This chapter summarizes the clinical drug-drug interaction data for each antiretroviral agent. The effects of antiretroviral agents on the pharmacokinetics of co-administered drugs will be discussed:

Nonnucleoside reverse transcriptase inhibitors (NNRTIs): delavirdine, efavirenz, etravirine, nevirapine, and rilpivirine

Nucleoside reverse-transcriptase inhibitors (NRTIs): abacavir, didanosine, emtricitabine, lamivudine, stavudine, tenofovir, and zidovudine

Protease inhibitors (PIs): atazanavir, darunavir, fosamprenavir, indinavir, nelfinavir, ritonavir, saquinavir, tipranavir, and lopinavir

Fusion inhibitors: enfuvirtide

Entry inhibitors: maraviroc

Integrase inhibitors: dolutegravir, elvitegravir, raltegravir

Methodology: A systematic literature search on PubMed and Google Scholar was conducted and the results cross-referenced with the prescribing information published by each manufacturer (as part of the FDA drug approval process) and Guidelines for the Use of Antiretroviral Agents in HIV-1-Infected Adults and Adolescent (AIDS info) published by the National Institutes of Health Research (Expert Guidelines) [1]. Only interactions supported by actual human data are presented in this chapter, and theoretically possible interactions are omitted.

T.K.L. Kiang • M.H.H. Ensom (✉)
Faculty of Pharmaceutical Sciences, The University of British Columbia, Vancouver, BC, Canada
e-mail: tkiang@gmail.com; mary.ensom@ubc.ca

K.J. Wilby
College of Pharmacy, Qatar University, Doha, Qatar
e-mail: kjw@qu.edu.qa

© Springer Science+Business Media Singapore 2016   79
T.K.L. Kiang et al. (eds.), *Pharmacokinetic and Pharmacodynamic Drug Interactions Associated with Antiretroviral Drugs*,
DOI 10.1007/978-981-10-2113-8_6

6.1   Nonnucleoside Reverse Transcriptase Inhibitors (NNRTIs)

6.1.1   *Delavirdine* (Table 6.1)

6.1.1.1   Analgesics

The effects of delavirdine on the pharmacokinetics of buprenorphine in opioid-dependent, non-HIV-infected subjects were determined by McCance-Katz et al. [2]. Under steady-state conditions, delavirdine increased the AUC and Cmax, but not the Cmin of buprenorphine. These effects were correlated with a ~75 % decrease in the apparent oral clearance (CL/F) of buprenorphine (Table 6.1). Consistent with these findings, delavirdine significantly decreased the clearance of norbuprenorphine metabolite (product of oxidation) but had little effect toward the glucuronide. Because delavirdine is a known inhibitor of CYP3A4 [3] and undergoes extensive oxidation via CYP3A4 [4], these findings suggest that delavirdine caused the significant pharmacokinetic interaction via CYP3A4 inhibition. However, it is not clear if the pharmacokinetic interaction is clinically relevant, as little changes in pharmacodynamics effects were reported in these subjects.

Table 6.1 Effects of delavirdine on the pharmacokinetics of co-administered drugs [2, 5, 7, 9–11, 15]

Drug	Summary effects on pharmacokinetics	Reference
Buprenorphine	↑ AUC (4.2×), ↑ Cmax (3.4×), ↓ Vd/F (75 %), ↓ CL/F (75 %)	McCance-Katz 2006
Clarithromycin	↑ AUC (1×), no change in Cmax	FDA clinical pharmacology document for delavirdine
Didanosine	No change in pharmacokinetic parameters	Morse 1997
Fluconazole	↑ AUC (1.3×), ↑ Cmax (2.8×), ↓ CL/F (22 %)	Borin 1997
Indinavir	↑ AUC (53 %), (with higher dose of indinavir), ↑ Cmax (36–53 %), ↑ Cmin (118–300 %)	Ferry 1998
Nelfinavir	↑ AUC (107 %), ↑ Cmax (98 %), ↑ Cmin (136 %)	FDA document
Rifabutin	No change in AUC, Cmax, tmax, CL/F, and t1/2	Borin 1997
Rifampin	No change in AUC, Cmax, tmax, CL/F, and t1/2	Borin 1997
Saquinavir	↑ AUC (121 %), ↑ Cmax (98 %), ↑ Cmin (199 %)	FDA document
Zidovudine	No change in pharmacokinetic parameters	FDA document

AUC area-under-the curve, *CL/F* apparent oral clearance, *Cmax* maximum concentration, *Cmin* minimum concentration, *t1/2* half-life, *tmax* time to maximal concentration, *Vd/F* apparent volume of distribution

6.1.1.2 Antimicrobials

The effects of delavirdine on the pharmacokinetics of various antimicrobials have been tested in humans. When clarithromycin (500 mg orally twice daily) was co-administered with delavirdine (300 mg orally twice daily) under steady-state conditions, the AUC of clarithromycin was increased (100%), but its Cmax remained the same [5]. These findings are consistent with the known metabolic properties of clarithromycin (a CYP3A4 substrate) [6] and delavirdine (a CYP3A4 inhibitor), but it is unclear whether the pharmacokinetic interaction resulted in altered pharmacodynamic characteristics (not tested). Moreover, the lack of information on other pharmacokinetic parameters such as CL/F and volume of distribution (Vd/F) precludes further mechanistic clarification regarding the nature of the observed interaction.

These findings are congruent with the results from an experiment where delavirdine (300 mg orally three times daily) was co-administered with another CYP3A4 substrate, fluconazole (400 mg orally once daily), under steady-state conditions in HIV-infected individuals ($N=13$) [7]. In this study, delavirdine increased the AUC (30%) and Cmax (180%) but decreased the CL/F (22%) of fluconazole, supporting a significant pharmacokinetic interaction between these agents. The findings from these two studies suggest that delavirdine, a known inhibitor of CYP3A4, can have significant effects on the pharmacokinetics of co-administered drugs metabolized by the same enzyme. However, because delavirdine is capable of inhibiting other CYP450 enzymes [8], pharmacokinetic interactions mediated by these other metabolic pathways should also be considered in delavirdine mediated drug-drug interactions.

In contrast to the finding of significant drug interactions mediated by delavirdine on the pharmacokinetics of CYP3A4 inhibitors (fluconazole/clarithromycin), significant changes in the pharmacokinetics of rifabutin or rifampin (CYP3A4 inducers) in the presence of delavirdine have not been observed. In HIV-infected subjects, delavirdine did not affect any measured pharmacokinetic parameters of rifabutin (300 mg orally once daily, $N=12$) or rifampin (600 mg orally once daily, $N=12$) under steady-state conditions [9, 10]. Because the co-administration of delavirdine with both agents is already contraindicated (due to significant changes in delavirdine pharmacokinetics, Chap. 5), the lack of significant alterations in the pharmacokinetics of rifampin or rifabutin still does not support the co-administration of these agents.

6.1.1.3 Protease Inhibitors

Data are available on the effects of delavirdine on the pharmacokinetics of indinavir, nelfinavir, and saquinavir [5]. Steady-state delavirdine (400 mg orally three times daily) significantly increased the Cmax, AUC, and Cmin of indinavir (to varying degrees of increase based on dose) given orally as single doses of 400, 600, or 800 mg in healthy subjects ($N=14$) [11]. Similarly, delavirdine was able to significantly increase the Cmax (98%), AUC (107% and 121%, respectively), and

Cmin (136 % and 199 %, respectively) of nelfinavir and saquinavir in healthy volunteers or subjects infected with HIV. These findings are consistent with the inhibitory effects of delavirdine toward the various CYP450 enzymes known to metabolize indinavir (CYP3A4) [12], nelfinavir (CYP3A4 and CYP2C19) [13], and saquinavir (CYP3A4) [14]. These results also indicate the suitability for using delavirdine to boost the effects of the tested protease inhibitors (hence "dose sparing").

6.1.1.4   Nucleoside Reverse Transcriptase Inhibitors

The effects of delavirdine on the pharmacokinetics of didanosine and zidovudine have been characterized in humans. Morse et al. [15] demonstrated that a single dose of delavirdine (400 mg) had little effect on the Cmax and AUC of didanosine (125–200 mg tablet) in HIV-infected patients ($N=12$). Likewise, steady-state delavirdine (400 mg orally three times daily) had no effect on the pharmacokinetic parameters of steady-state zidovudine (200 mg orally three times daily, $N=42$). These findings are likely the result of the nonoverlapping metabolic characteristics of delavirdine (primarily metabolized by CYP3A4) and zidovudine (primarily conjugated by UGT enzymes) [16] or didanosine (purine-like degradation) in humans (Chap. 4).

6.1.2   *Efavirenz* (Table 6.2)

6.1.2.1   Analgesics

The effects of efavirenz on the pharmacokinetics of buprenorphine in opioid-dependent, non-HIV-infected subjects were determined by McCance-Katz et al. [2]. Under steady-state conditions, efavirenz decreased the AUC and Cmax, but not the Cmin of buprenorphine. These effects were correlated with a ~twofold increase in the CL/F of buprenorphine (Table 6.2). Consistent with these findings, efavirenz significantly reduced the exposure of the norbuprenorphine metabolite (product of oxidation) and the glucuronide, which is consistent with the known CYP3A4 induction properties of efavirenz [17]. The significant reduction in norbuprenorphine plasma concentrations is contradictory to the hypothesized CYP3A4 induction effects of efavirenz, but indicates that other enzyme pathways may be involved in this drug interaction. Similar to buprenorphine, steady-state efavirenz (500 mg orally daily) decreased the Cmax (45 %) and AUC (52 %) of subjects maintained on stable doses of methadone (35–100 mg/day) [18]. Because methadone is known to be metabolized by CYP3A4 [19] and efavirenz is documented to be a potent CYP3A4 inducer, the significant pharmacokinetic interaction observed is likely also mediated by this enzyme. It is unclear if the N-demethylated metabolite of

Table 6.2 Effects of efavirenz on the pharmacokinetics of co-administered drugs [2, 18, 21, 22, 24, 26, 28–31]

Drug	Summary effects on pharmacokinetics	Reference
Artemether/lumefantrine	↓ artemether AUC (51–78 %) No change in lumefantrine AUC in healthy subjects; ↓ 55 % in HIV patients. day-7 level ↓ (46 %) in healthy subjects	Huang 2012 Byakika-Kibwika
Atovaquone/proguanil	↓ atovaquone AUC (75 %), ↓ proguanil AUC (38–43 %)	van Luin 2010
Atorvastatin	↓ AUC (43 %)	Gerber 2005
Azithromycin	No change on AUC, ↑ Cmax (22 %)	FDA document
Buprenorphine	↓ AUC (49 %), ↓ Cmax (45 %), ↑ CL/F (2.1×)	McCance-Katz 2006
Bupropion	↓ AUC (55 %)	Robertson 2008
Carbamazepine	↓ AUC (27 %)	Ji 2008
Clarithromycin	↓ AUC (39 %), ↓ Cmax (26 %)	FDA document
Ethinyl estradiol	↑ AUC (37 %)	FDA document
Fluconazole	No change in pharmacokinetic parameters	FDA document
Lamivudine	No change in pharmacokinetic parameters	FDA document
Levonorgestrel	↓ AUC (56 %), ↓ Cmax (41 %)	Carten 2012
Lopinavir/ritonavir	↓ AUC (19 %)	FDA document
Methadone	↓ AUC (52 %), ↓ Cmax (45 %)	FDA document
Nelfinavir	↑ AUC (20 %), ↑ Cmax (21 %)	FDA document
Paroxetine	No change in pharmacokinetic parameters	FDA document
Pravastatin	↓ AUC (40 %)	Gerber 2005
Rifabutin	↓ AUC (38 %), ↓ Cmax (32 %)	FDA document
Ritonavir	↑ AUC (18 %), ↑ Cmax (24 %)	FDA document
Saquinavir	↓ AUC (62 %), ↓ Cmax (50 %)	FDA document
Sertraline	↓ AUC (39 %), ↓ Cmax (29 %)	FDA document
Simvastatin	↓ AUC (58 %)	Gerber 2005
Tipranavir/ritonavir	No change in pharmacokinetics parameters	la Prote 2009
Voriconazole	↓AUC (77 %), ↓ Cmax (61 %)	FDA document
Zidovudine	No change in pharmacokinetic parameters	FDA document

AUC area-under-the curve, *Cmax* maximum concentration

methadone was characterized in this study, which would have provided more definitive data in support of the proposed interaction. Overall, these data suggest that the co-administration of efavirenz in individuals maintained on buprenorphine and methadone may potentially decrease the drugs' efficacy, resulting in manifestation of withdrawal effects.

6.1.2.2 Antimicrobials

The effects of efavirenz on the pharmacokinetics of several antimicrobial agents (azithromycin, clarithromycin, fluconazole, rifabutin, rifampin, and voriconazole) have been characterized in humans [18]. For the macrolides, steady-state efavirenz did not have a significant effect on the exposure of azithromycin given at a single dose (600 mg, $N = 14$). This is in contrast to the findings obtained with the other macrolide (500 mg orally twice daily) where steady-state efavirenz (400 mg orally daily, $N = 11$) decreased both the Cmax (26 %) and the AUC (39 %) of clarithromycin, with corresponding increases in the exposure of the 14-hydroxymetabolite. These findings are in agreement with the induction of CYP3A4 by efavirenz, which resulted in increased intrinsic clearance of clarithromycin. The discrepant findings between clarithromycin and azithromycin may be explained by the fact that CYP3A4 is the primary enzyme responsible for the oxidation of clarithromycin but contributes only to a minor extent in the metabolism of azithromycin. Taken together with the observation that neither macrolide affected efavirenz exposure (Chap. 5) and that efavirenz had minimal effect on the pharmacokinetics of azithromycin, azithromycin would be considered the drug of choice (over clarithromycin) if a macrolide antibiotic is required for the treatment of infections in patients taking efavirenz.

Differential effects on the pharmacokinetics of fluconazole and voriconazole from the co-administration of efavirenz were observed in humans [18]. Under steady-state conditions, efavirenz (400 mg orally daily) did not affect the Cmax or the AUC of fluconazole (200 mg orally daily, $N = 10$). This is in contrast to the significant reductions in voriconazole (400 mg orally every 12 h) Cmax (61 %) and AUC (77 %) when efavirenz (400 mg orally daily) was co-administered under steady-state conditions. The differences in the degree of pharmacokinetic interactions may be due to the inductive effects of efavirenz toward CYP3A4, which may play a more prominent role in voriconazole metabolism compared with that of fluconazole. The lack of pharmacokinetic interactions between fluconazole and efavirenz and the significant interactions observed between voriconazole and efavirenz suggest that fluconazole should be used (over voriconazole) for patients taking efavirenz if an azole antifungal is needed for the treatment of infections.

The effects of efavirenz on the pharmacokinetics of rifabutin have also been characterized in humans, where steady-state efavirenz (600 mg orally daily) significantly reduced the Cmax (32 %) and AUC (38 %) of steady-state rifabutin (300 mg orally daily, $N = 9$) [18]. Because rifabutin is primarily metabolized by CYP3A4 [20], these data confirm the potent inductive effects of efavirenz on this enzyme as the likely mechanism of the interaction. One might also hypothesize that efavirenz is a more potent CYP3A4 inducer than rifabutin, which is supported by the observation that efavirenz decreased rifabutin exposure, but not vice versa. The potency of CYP3A4 induction by efavirenz has been hypothesized to be on par to that of rifampin (Chap. 4).

6.1.2.3 HMG-CoA Inhibitors

The effects of efavirenz on the pharmacokinetics of simvastatin, atorvastatin, and pravastatin have been characterized in healthy volunteers ($N=52$) [21]. Efavirenz (600 mg orally daily) was able to significantly decrease the AUC of simvastatin (58%), atorvastatin (43%), and pravastatin (40%), under steady-state conditions. The reduced exposure of simvastatin corresponded with suppressed HMG-CoA reductase inhibition, highlighting a significant pharmacokinetic-pharmacodynamic relationship based on the drug interaction. Because these statins are all primarily metabolized by CYP3A4, the most likely underlying mechanism for the interaction is enzyme induction from efavirenz. Based on these findings, the lipid lowering effects of HMG-CoA inhibitors might be reduced in the presence of efavirenz, and alternative statins, such as rosuvastatin, which do not undergo CYP3A4-mediated oxidation, may be better choices in this setting.

6.1.2.4 Miscellaneous Agents

The effects of efavirenz on the pharmacokinetics of bupropion, carbamazepine, ethinyl estradiol, levonorgestrel, paroxetine, and sertraline have been characterized in humans. Steady-state efavirenz significantly reduced the AUC (55%) of a single dose bupropion (sustained-release 150 mg) in healthy subjects ($N=13$) and increased the hydroxybupropion metabolite to bupropion ratio by ~2.3-fold [22]. Because bupropion is primarily oxidized by CYP2B6 [23], these findings indicate a significant induction effect by efavirenz toward this specific enzyme.

In healthy subjects receiving steady-state efavirenz (600 mg orally daily) and carbamazepine (400 mg orally daily), the AUC (27%) of carbamazepine was significantly reduced in the presence of efavirenz [24]. The induction of CYP3A4 (the primary enzymes responsible for carbamazepine metabolism) [25] by efavirenz is the proposed mechanism underlying the interaction, although metabolite analysis to characterize altered intrinsic clearance (i.e. increased carbamazepine epoxide formation) is needed to confirm this hypothesis. Although it is unclear if altered pharmacokinetics would result in a clinically significant reduction in carbamazepine efficacy, these findings suggest that alternative antiseizure pharmacotherapy other than carbamazepine should be considered when used in combination with efavirenz.

Different effects of efavirenz on the pharmacokinetics of hormone contraceptives have been documented in humans. Steady-state efavirenz (400–600 mg orally daily, $N=13$) increased the AUC of a single 50 μg ethinyl estradiol dose by ~37% [18], but decreased the Cmax (41%) and AUC (56%) of levonorgestrel (0.75 mg) [26]. The effects of efavirenz on the pharmacokinetics of levonorgestrel are likely mediated by CYP3A4 induction, but it is not clear why a similar interaction was not observed with ethinyl estradiol as both hormones are primarily metabolized by CYP3A4. These contradictory findings may be the result of the mixed inhibitory/induction characteristics exhibit by efavirenz, although further metabolism studies are needed to confirm this hypothesis. Based on these results, failure of contraception may be possible when efavirenz is co-administered.

Steady-state efavirenz (600 mg orally daily) also exhibited different effects on the pharmacokinetics of steady-state paroxetine (20 mg orally daily) and sertraline (50 mg orally daily, $N = 12$–13) [18]. Efavirenz did not affect the pharmacokinetics of paroxetine but decreased the Cmax (29%) and AUC (39%) of sertraline. The findings with paroxetine are consistent with its metabolic properties that lacked interaction potential with the known metabolic pathways of efavirenz. On the other hand, efavirenz is yet not known to induce CYP2D6 or CYP2C19, enzymes known for the oxidation of sertraline [27]; thus, alternative mechanisms (i.e. unidentified metabolic pathways of either agent) may be responsible.

6.1.2.5   Antimalarials

The effects of efavirenz on the pharmacokinetics of artemether/lumefantrine and atovaquone/plaquenil have been investigated in humans. In healthy volunteers ($N = 12$), efavirenz (600 mg orally daily for 26 days) significantly decreased the AUC (51%) of artemether (80 mg orally twice daily) but not lumefantrine (480 mg orally twice daily, in combination with artemether) [28]. However, the day 7 lumefantrine concentration, typically designated as a surrogate marker for therapeutic activity, was significantly reduced (46%) by efavirenz co-administration. These changes also corresponded with decreased exposure of the active metabolite of artemether (dihydroartemisinin), which may potentially lead to decreased therapeutic efficacy of artemether/lumefantrine. Similar findings were also observed in HIV-infected adults [29], where steady-state efavirenz therapy decreased the AUC (78% and 55%) of both artemether and lumefantrine (steady-state dosing of 80 mg/480 mg twice daily $\times$ 3 days), respectively. The mechanism of interaction is likely efavirenz-mediated induction of CYP3A4, which is the primary enzyme responsible for the oxidation of both artemether and lumefantrine.

The exposure of atovaquone and plaquenil in HIV-infected patients taking efavirenz has been compared to that in healthy subjects taking atovaquone/plaquanil alone [30]. Although this experiment was not adequately controlled, the HIV-infected patients (co-administered efavirenz) had significantly lower AUCs of atovaquone ($\downarrow$75%) and plaquenil ($\downarrow$43%) compared to healthy subjects not taking efavirenz. These data appear to support an inductive effect of efavirenz on the metabolism of atovaquone/plaquanil, but the known metabolic characteristics do not support a mechanistic interaction between these agents. The observed apparent interaction between these agents may be the result of the inadequate control or the involvement of alternative metabolic pathways that have not yet been characterized for these drugs.

6.1.2.6   Antivirals

Differential effects of efavirenz on the pharmacokinetics of various protease inhibitors (lopinavir/ritonavir, nelfinavir, ritonavir, saquinavir, and tipranavir/ritonavir) have been characterized in humans. Steady-state efavirenz (600 mg orally daily) demonstrated the following significant effects: decreased the AUC (19 %) of steady-state lopinavir (400 mg in conjunction with ritonavir 100 mg orally every 12 h, $N=11$); increased the Cmax (21 %) and AUC (20 %) of nelfinavir (750 mg orally every 8 h, $N=10$) with corresponding decreased exposure of the nelfinavir metabolite; increased the Cmax (21 %) and AUC (18 %) of ritonavir (500 mg orally every 12 h, $N=11$); decreased the Cmax (50 %) and AUC (62 %) of saquinavir (1200 mg orally every 8 h, $N=12$); and did not change the pharmacokinetics of tipranavir/ritonavir (500 mg/200 mg orally twice daily, $N=34$) [18, 31]. Decreased lopinavir and saquinavir exposure from the co-administration of efavirenz corresponds to the tendency of efavirenz to induce CYP3A4, which is responsible for the metabolism of these antivirals. On the other hand, the apparent higher exposure values of nelfinavir or ritonavir and the lack of change in the pharmacokinetics of tipranavir are difficult to explain. These contradictory observations may be due to the mixed inhibitory/induction effects of efavirenz toward various CYP450 enzyme systems; however, the exact mechanisms are difficult to determine in clinical experiments and better suited for in vitro mechanistic investigations.

The effects of efavirenz on the metabolism of nucleoside reverse transcriptase inhibitors have been characterized in humans [18]. Efavirenz (600 mg orally daily) did not change the pharmacokinetics of lamivudine (150 mg orally every 12 h) or zidovudine (300 mg orally every 12 h) under steady-state conditions ($N=9$). Because lamivudine is not extensively metabolized and zidovudine primarily undergoes UGT-mediated conjugation, the lack of drug interaction with efavirenz is consistent with the nonoverlapping metabolism characteristics between these agents.

6.1.3 *Etravirine* (Table 6.3)

6.1.3.1 Antimalarial

The effects of steady-state (200 mg orally twice daily) etravirine co-administration on the pharmacokinetics of a 3-day treatment course of artemether/lumefantrine (80 mg/480 mg) were determined in healthy subjects ($N=33$) [32]. Etravirine significantly decreased the AUCs of both artemether (38 %) and lumefantrine (13 %), which corresponded with decreased dihydroartemisinin (active metabolite of artemether) exposure of 15 %. These data support the potent induction effects of etravirine toward CYP3A4, the primary enzyme responsible for the oxidation of artemether/lumefantrine, and perhaps the subsequent glucuronidation of dihydroartemisinin. However, the latter effect requires further confirmation, because relatively little data are available supporting an induction effect of etravirine toward the UGT enzymes. Based on these findings, etravirine may potentially reduce the efficacy of artemether/lumefantrine; therefore, their co-administration is not recommended.

Table 6.3 Effects of etravirine on the pharmacokinetics of co-administered drugs [32, 33, 35]

Drug	Summary effects on pharmacokinetics	Reference
Artemether/lumefantrine	↓ artemether AUC (38 %) ↓ lumefantrine AUC (13 %)	Kakuda 2013
Atazanavir	↓ AUC (17 %), ↓ Cmin (47 %)	FDA document
Atazanavir/ritonavir	↓ AUC (14 %)	FDA document
Atorvastatin	↓ AUC (43 %)	FDA document
Boceprevir	↑ AUC (10 %)	Hammond 2013
Clarithromycin	↓ AUC (39 %), ↓ Cmax (34 %)	FDA document
Darunavir/ritonavir	No significant change in pharmacokinetic parameters for darunavir	FDA document
Didanosine	No significant change in pharmacokinetic parameters	FDA document
Ethinyl estradiol	↑ AUC (22 %), ↑ Cmax (33 %)	FDA document
Fosamprenavir/ritonavir	↑ AUC (69 %), ↑ Cmax (62 %)	FDA document
Lopinavir/ritonavir	↓ lopinavir AUC (20 %)	FDA document
R(−), S(+) Methadone	No significant change in pharmacokinetic parameters	FDA document
Norethindrone	No significant change in pharmacokinetic parameters	FDA document
Paroxetine	No significant change in pharmacokinetic parameters	FDA document
Raltegravir	No significant change in pharmacokinetic parameters	FDA document
Rifabutin	↓ AUC (17 %)	FDA document
Saquinavir/ritonavir	No significant change in pharmacokinetic parameters	FDA document
Sildenafil	↓ AUC (57 %), ↓ Cmax (45 %)	FDA document
Tenofovir	No significant change in pharmacokinetic parameters	FDA document
Tipranavir/ritonavir	↑ tipranavir AUC (18 %), ↑ Cmax (14 %)	FDA document

AUC area-under-the curve, *Cmax* maximum concentration, *Cmin* minimum concentration

6.1.3.2 Antimicrobials

The effects of etravirine on the pharmacokinetics of clarithromycin and rifabutin have been reported. Etravirine significantly decreased the Cmax (34 %) and AUC (39 %) of clarithromycin (500 mg orally twice daily, $N = 15$) with corresponding increases in the Cmax and AUC of its primary metabolite, 14-hydroxy-clarithromycin [33]. On the other hand, etravirine decreased the AUCs of both rifabutin (17 %) and its metabolite, 25-O-desacetylrifabutin, without having much effect on other pharmacokinetic parameters. The effects of etravirine on clarithromycin and rifabutin pharmacokinetics corresponded with the known inductive effects of etravirine on CYP3A4 [34], the primary enzyme responsible for the hydroxylation of clarithromycin and deacetylation of rifabutin. The characterization of 14-hydroxy-clarithromycin also provides confirmatory data supporting the increase of clarithromycin intrinsic clearance as the mechanism responsible for the observed interaction. On the other hand, reduction of 25-O-desacetyl-rifabutin concentration might indicate that efavirenz may have also induced subsequent metabolism of the metabolite (hence further increasing degradation), but this hypothesis remains to be tested.

6.1.3.3   Miscellaneous Agents

The effects of etravirine on the pharmacokinetics of atorvastatin, boceprevir, ethinyl estradiol, methadone, norethindrone, paroxetine, and sildenafil have been characterized in humans [33, 35]. Steady-state etravirine significantly reduced the AUCs (43 % and 57 %) of atorvastatin (40 mg orally daily, $N = 16$) and sildenafil (50 mg single dose, $N = 15$), respectively. These findings corresponded with increased 2-hydroxy-atorvastatin exposure but decreased N-desmethyl-sildenafil concentration [33]. Etravirine likely increased the metabolism of atorvastatin and enhanced the formation of 2-hydroxy-atorvastatin by the induction of CYP3A4, the primary enzyme responsible for the hydroxylation of atorvastatin [36]. On the other hand, sildenafil is also metabolized by CYP3A4 [37]; thus, the decreased sildenafil AUC may also be mediated by CYP3A4 induction. However, it is unclear how etravirine co-administration resulted in decreased N-desmethyl-sildenafil formation. The potential induction of subsequent pathways of N-desmethyl-sildenafil metabolism by etravirine may be possible and warrants further mechanistic investigation. On the other hand, etravirine modestly increased the AUC of ethinyl estradiol (22 %) and boceprevir (10 %), but had little effects toward the pharmacokinetics of norethindrone, methadone, and paroxetine. It is difficult to ascertain the mechanisms of these interactions based on the known metabolic characteristics of these drugs. The modest observed effects (i.e., with ethinyl estradiol and boceprevir) may also not translate to clinically relevant pharmacodynamic effects. Further studies in larger populations are warranted to confirm these observations.

6.1.3.4   Protease Inhibitors

Mixed effects of etravirine toward the pharmacokinetics of various protease inhibitors (atazanavir, atazanavir/ritonavir, darunavir/ritonavir, fosamprenavir/ritonavir, lopinavir/ritonavir, saquinavir/ritonavir, and tipranavir/ritonavir) have been characterized. Steady-state etravirine significantly decreased the AUCs of atazanavir (14–17 %, 400 mg orally daily or in combination with ritonavir 100 mg) and lopinavir (20 %, 400 mg with 100 mg ritonavir twice daily) in humans [33]. On the other hand, etravirine did not alter the pharmacokinetics of darunavir (darunavir/ritonavir, 600 mg/100 mg twice daily) and saquinavir (saquinavir/ritonavir, 1000 mg/100 mg twice daily), but significantly increased the AUCs of amprenavir (69 %, fosamprenavir/ritonavir, 700 mg/100 mg twice daily) and tipranavir (18 %, tipranavir/ritonavir). The apparently decreased exposures of ata-zanavir and lopinavir may be explained by the induction effects of etravirine toward CYP3A4, the primary enzyme responsible for the oxidation of these sub-strates (Chap. 4). On the other hand, the lack of effects of etravirine toward darunavir or saquinavir pharmacokinetics and the apparently increased exposures of amprenavir and tipranavir from etravirine co-administration may be due to interference from the pharmacological boosting agent ritonavir, which is itself a potent inhibitor of various CYP450 enzymes. Consequently, these observations may be the result of complex metabolic interactions mediated by opposing enzyme inhibition or induction activities.

6.1.3.5 Nucleoside Reverse Transcriptase Inhibitors and Integrase Inhibitors

The ability of etravirine to alter the pharmacokinetics of didanosine (400 mg orally daily), tenofovir (300 mg orally daily), and raltegravir (400 mg orally twice daily) has been characterized in humans [33]. No significant interactions with didanosine, tenofovir, and raltegravir from etravirine co-administration were observed in these studies, which support the general lack of metabolism-mediated drug interaction potential of didanosine and the nonoverlapping meta-bolic pathways between raltegravir, tenofovir, and etravirine (Chap. 4). The lack of bidirectional interactions between these antiretrovirals (see Chap. 5) suggests that their co-administration would not result in significant pharmacodynamic interactions.

6.1.4   Nevirapine (Table 6.4)

6.1.4.1   Antimalarial

The effects of steady-state nevirapine co-administration on the pharmacokinetics of a 3-day treatment course of artemether/lumefantrine (80 mg/480 mg) were deter-mined in HIV-infected subjects [29]. Nevirapine significantly decreased the AUC of artemether (72 %), which corresponded with decreased dihydroartemisinin (active metabolite of artemether) exposure (37 %). These data support the induction effects of nevirapine on CYP3A4, the primary enzyme responsible for the oxidation of artemether, and perhaps the subsequent glucuronidation of dihydroartemisinin. However, the latter effect requires further confirmation, because little is known about the activities of nevirapine toward the UGT enzymes. On the other hand, nevi-rapine did not alter the pharmacokinetics of lumefantrine, which may be due to the relatively weaker induction effects of nevirapine toward CYP3A4 compared to other NNRTIs (e.g., etravirine) which have been known to reduce the exposure of lumefantrine [32].

Table 6.4 Effects of nevirapine on the pharmacokinetics of co-administered drugs [29, 38, 39]

Drug	Summary effects on pharmacokinetics	Reference
Artemether/lumefantrine	↓ artemether AUC (72 %) No change to lumefantrine pharmacokinetics	Byakika-Kibwika 2012
Atazanavir/ritonavir	↓ AUC (42 %), ↓ Cmax (28 %)	FDA document
Buprenorphine	No significant change in pharmacokinetic parameters	McCance-Katz 2010
Clarithromycin	↓ AUC (31 %), ↓ Cmax (23 %)	FDA document
Darunavir/ritonavir	↑ AUC (24 %), ↑ Cmax (40 %)	FDA document
Didanosine	No significant change in pharmacokinetic parameters	FDA document
Ethinyl estradiol	↓ AUC (20 %)	FDA document
Fluconazole	No significant change in pharmacokinetic parameters	FDA document
Fosamprenavir/ritonavir	↓ AUC (11 %)	FDA document
Fosamprenavir	↓ AUC (33 %), ↓ Cmax (25 %)	FDA document
Indinavir	↓ AUC (31 %), ↓ Cmax (15 %)	FDA document
Ketoconazole	↓ AUC (72 %), ↓ Cmax (44 %)	FDA document
Lopinavir/ritonavir	↓ AUC (27 %), ↓ Cmax (19 %)	FDA document
Maraviroc	↑ AUC (1 %) [please verify!!], ↑ Cmax (54 %)	FDA document
Methadone	↓ AUC (37–51 %), ↑ clearance 3×	FDA document
Nelfinavir	No significant change in pharmacokinetic parameters	FDA document
Norethindrone	↓ AUC (19 %), ↓ Cmax (16 %)	FDA document
Rifabutin	↑ AUC (17 %), ↑ Cmax (28 %)	FDA document
Rifampin	↑ AUC (11 %), no change in Cmax	FDA document
Ritonavir	No significant change in pharmacokinetic parameters	FDA document
Stavudine	No significant change in pharmacokinetic parameters	FDA document
Zidovudine	↓ AUC (28 %), ↓ Cmax (30 %)	FDA document

AUC area-under-the curve, *Cmax* maximum concentration

6.1.4.2   Analgesics

The effects of nevirapine on the pharmacokinetics of buprenorphine in opioid-dependent, non-HIV-infected subjects [38] and the pharmacokinetics of methadone in HIV-infected patients [39] have been characterized. Under steady-state conditions, nevirapine (200 mg orally daily) did not affect the AUC of buprenorphine or its metabolites, with a modest increase (not statistically significant) in the clearance of buprenorphine. These effects are consistent with the relatively weak (i.e., nonsignificant) induction potency of nevirapine toward CYP3A4, in contrast to other NNRTIs (e.g., efavirenz) that are relatively more potent enzyme inducers which have been correlated with significantly increased oral clearance of buprenorphine.

The lack of significant effects on pharmacokinetics corresponds with the minimal changes in the pharmacodynamic effects of buprenorphine.

In contrast to buprenorphine, steady-state nevirapine (200 mg orally daily, $N=9$) decreased the Cmax (37–51 %) and increased the oral clearance of methadone (~2×) in HIV-infected subjects already on stable doses of the opioid analgesic [39]. The significant pharmacokinetic changes corresponded with withdrawal effects in the majority of subjects enrolled in the study, confirming a pharmacokinetic-pharmacodynamic interaction. Because methadone is known to be metabolized by CYP3A4 and nevirapine is a documented CYP3A4 inducer, the significant pharmacokinetic interaction observed is likely mediated by this enzyme. However, it is unclear why nevirapine (a relatively weak inducer of CYP3A4) was capable of inducing a significant pharmacokinetic interaction with methadone but not buprenorphine (also primarily metabolized by the same enzyme). Perhaps the effects of nevirapine toward other metabolic enzymes responsible for buprenorphine metabolism may have contributed to these findings. Overall, these data suggest that the co-administration of efavirenz in individuals maintained on methadone may potentially decrease the opioid's efficacy and result in the manifestation of withdrawal effects.

6.1.4.3   Antimicrobials

The effects of nevirapine on the pharmacokinetics of several antimicrobial agents (clarithromycin, fluconazole, ketoconazole, rifabutin, and rifampin) have been characterized in humans [39]. Steady-state nevirapine (200 mg orally daily) significantly decreased the Cmax (23 %) and AUC (31 %) of clarithromycin (500 mg orally twice daily, $N=15$), with corresponding increases in the exposure of 14-hydroxy-clarithromycin (42 %). These findings are in agreement with the induction of CYP3A4 by nevirapine, leading to increased intrinsic clearance of clarithromycin (primarily metabolized by CYP3A4) and increased formation of its hydroxylated metabolite. In contrast to other NNRTIs, the effects of nevirapine on azithromycin pharmacokinetics have not been tested in humans. Thus, it remains to be determined if azithromycin remains a better option than clarithromycin (as for other NNRTI combinations discussed above) if a macrolide is needed in conjunction with nevirapine.

Differential effects on the pharmacokinetics of fluconazole and ketoconazole from the co-administration of nevirapine have been documented in humans [39]. Under steady-state conditions, nevirapine (200 mg orally daily) did not affect the Cmax or AUC of fluconazole (200 mg orally daily, $N=19$), which is in contrast to the significant reductions in ketoconazole (400 mg orally daily) Cmax (44 %) and AUC (72 %) when nevirapine (200 mg orally daily) was co-administered under steady-state conditions in HIV-infected patients. The differences in the degree of pharmacokinetic interactions may be due to the inductive effects of nevirapine toward CYP3A4, which may play a more prominent role in ketoconazole metabolism than fluconazole. Even though nevirapine did not change the pharmacokinetics of fluconazole, fluconazole appeared to be capable of increasing the exposure of nevirapine (Chap. 5). Based on these findings, the co-administration of fluconazole with these azole antifungals would not be recommended.

The effects of nevirapine on the pharmacokinetics of rifabutin or rifampin have been characterized in humans. Steady-state nevirapine (200 mg orally daily) significantly increased the Cmax (17%, no change for rifampin) and AUC (17% and 11%) of steady-state rifabutin (150 or 300 mg orally daily, $N=19$) and rifampin (600 mg orally daily, $N=14$). [39]. The formation of 25-O-desacetyl-rifabutin was also increased as evident by increased Cmax (24%) and exposure (29%) in the presence of nevirapine. Because both rifabutin and rifampin are primarily metabolized by CYP3A4, these data are contradictory to the known inductive effects of nevirapine toward the same enzyme (Chap. 4). However, the degree of induction (based on % increase in AUC) appeared relatively small (11–17%); thus, it may be possible that these contradictory findings could be the result of random variability (especially from the small sample sizes), and more importantly, it is unclear whether these findings are clinically relevant.

6.1.4.4   Oral Contraceptives

Effects of nevirapine on the pharmacokinetics of hormone contraceptives have been documented in humans. Steady-state efavirenz (200 mg orally once or twice daily, $N=10$) decreased the AUCs (19–20%) of steady-state ethinyl estradiol (0.035 mg) and norethindrone (1 mg, given in combination with ethinyl estradiol) [39]. The effects of nevirapine on the pharmacokinetics of levonorgestrel and norethindrone are likely mediated by CYP3A4 induction, as both hormones are primarily metabolized by the same enzyme. Based on these results, failure of contraception may be possible when nevirapine is co-administered.

6.1.4.5   Antiretrovirals

Mixed effects of nevirapine toward the pharmacokinetics of various protease inhibitors (atazanavir/ritonavir, darunavir/ritonavir, fosamprenavir/ritonavir, fosamprenavir, indinavir, lopinavir/ritonavir, nelfinavir, and ritonavir) have been characterized [39]. Steady-state nevirapine significantly decreased the AUCs of atazanavir (19–42%, 300–400 mg orally daily in combination with ritonavir 100 mg), amprenavir (11–33%, from fosamprenavir 1400 mg twice daily or fosamprenavir/ritonavir 700 mg/100 mg twice daily), indinavir (31%, 800 mg every 8 h), and lopinavir (22–27%, from 300 to 400 mg lopinavir with 100 mg ritonavir), increased the AUC of darunavir (24%, 400 mg darunavir with 100 mg ritonavir), and had little effect on the exposure of nelfinavir (750 mg three times daily, despite significantly decreased exposure of the metabolite) and ritonavir alone (600 mg twice daily). The decreased exposures of the mentioned protease inhibitors may be explained by the induction effects of nevirapine toward CYP3A4, the primary enzyme responsible for the oxidation of these substrates (Chap. 4). On the other hand, the lack of effects of nevirapine on nelfinavir or ritonavir pharmacokinetics and the apparently increased exposures of darunavir (boosted by ritonavir) co-administration may be difficult to explain, as these drugs are also primarily metabolized by CYP3A4. Interference from the pharmacological boosting agent ritonavir, which is itself a potent inhibitor of various CYP450 enzymes, may explain the apparently increased exposure of darunavir. Further mechanistic studies are required to determine the apparent lack of effects of nevirapine on nelfinavir or ritonavir metabolism.

The ability of nevirapine (200 mg orally daily) to alter the pharmacokinetics of NRTIs, didanosine (100–150 mg orally twice daily), stavudine (30–40 mg twice daily), and zidovudine (100–200 mg three times daily), has been characterized under steady-state conditions in HIV-infected subjects [39]. No significant interactions with didanosine and stavudine from nevirapine co-administration were observed in these studies, supporting the general lack of metabolism-mediated drug interaction potential of didanosine or stavudine (Chap. 4). On the other hand, nevirapine significantly decreased the Cmax (30%) and AUC (28%) of zidovudine ($N=11$), an effect not supported by the currently known metabolic properties of either agent; zidovudine is primarily conjugated by UGT enzymes that are not yet known to be modulated by nevirapine (Chap. 4). Moreover, the degree of induction (based on % increase in AUC) was relatively small (28%); thus, it may be possible that these contradictory findings could be the results of random variability from the small sample size used in this experiment. The general lack of bidirectional interactions between nevirapine and NRTIs (see Chap. 5) suggests that their co-administration would not result in significant pharmacodynamic interactions.

The effects of nevirapine on the pharmacokinetics of maraviroc, an entry inhibitor, have been characterized in HIV-infected patients [39]. Under steady-state conditions, nevirapine (200 mg orally twice daily, $N=8$) had very little effect on the exposure or Cmax of maraviroc, but these observations corresponded with relatively large variabilities reported for both pharmacokinetic parameters. The reported effects are not consistent with the known metabolism characteristics of maraviroc (primarily metabolized by CYP3A4) or nevirapine (an inducer of CYP3A4). However, because maraviroc is known to be subject to CYP3A4-mediated drug-drug interactions (Chap. 4), the lack of apparent interaction between these two agents might be explained by the relatively nonpotent induction properties of nevirapine. Further studies in larger sample populations are needed to characterize the interaction (or lack of) between these two agents.

6.1.5   *Rilpivirine* (Table 6.5)

The effects of rilpivirine on the pharmacokinetics of co-administered drugs have been characterized extensively by the manufacturer, but most of these experiments were conducted at relatively higher concentrations of rilpivirine (i.e., 75 mg or

Table 6.5   Effects of rilpivirine on the pharmacokinetics of co-administered drugs [40]

Drug	Summary effects on pharmacokinetics	Reference
Acetaminophen	No significant change in pharmacokinetic parameters	FDA document
Atorvastatin	No significant change in pharmacokinetic parameters	FDA document
Chlorzoxazone	No significant change in pharmacokinetic parameters	FDA document
Darunavir/ritonavir	No significant change in pharmacokinetic parameters	FDA document
Didanosine	No significant change in pharmacokinetic parameters	FDA document
Ethinyl estradiol	↑ AUC (14 %), ↑ Cmax (17 %)	FDA document
Ketoconazole	↓ AUC (24 %), ↓ Cmax (15 %)	FDA document
Lopinavir/ritonavir	No significant change in pharmacokinetic parameters	FDA document
R(−), S(+) Methadone	↓ AUC (16 %), ↓ Cmax (14 %)	FDA document
Norethindrone	No significant change in pharmacokinetic parameters	FDA document
Omeprazole	↓ AUC (14 %), ↓ Cmax (14 %)	FDA document
Rifampin	No significant change in pharmacokinetic parameters	FDA document
Sildenafil	No significant change in pharmacokinetic parameters	FDA document
Tenofovir	↑ AUC (23 %), ↑ Cmax (19 %)	FDA document

Most of the drug interaction studies summarized in this table have been conducted at suprathera-peutic dosing of rilpivirine and may not be clinically relevant (see text for details)

AUC area-under-the curve, *Cmax* maximum concentration

150 mg once daily), which have not been approved for therapeutic use (Table 6.5) [40]. As a result, these data would likely not be relevant for the clinic. On the other hand, steady-state rilpivirine (approved dosing of 25 mg daily) was shown to increase the AUC (14 %) and Cmax (17 %) of ethinyl estradiol (0.035 mg, given with norethindrone 1 mg) and decrease the AUC (11 %) of norethindrone ($N = 17$). Similar to the oral contraceptives, rilpivirine (approved dosing of 25 mg daily) modestly decreased the AUCs (~16 %) and Cmax (~13–14 %) of R(−) or S(+) methadone under steady-state conditions. The inhibitory effects of rilpivirine toward CYP3A4 [41] may be responsible for the elevation of ethinyl estradiol AUC, but further studies are needed to characterize the mechanisms associated with the apparent rilpivirine/norethindrone or rilpivirine/methadone interaction in humans. Although rilpivirine is known to induce CYP3A4 in cell lines (Chap. 4), these observations have not yet been confirmed in more conventional systems suitable for the study of drug-drug interactions (e.g., primary cultures of human hepatocytes). Overall, these modest effects would indicate that the interactions are likely not clinically relevant.

6.2   Nucleoside Reverse-Transcriptase Inhibitors (NRTIs)

6.2.1   *Abacavir* (Table 6.6)

Little information is available in the literature on metabolism-mediated drug-drug interactions associated with abacavir in humans, which is consistent with the fact that it is not a substrate of the CYP450 enzymes (Chap. 4). However, because abacavir undergoes conjugation by UGTs (the exact identities of the enzymes involved remain to be determined) [42], it can potentially inhibit (competitively) the conjugation of other co-administered drugs.

6.2.2   *Didanosine* (Table 6.7)

Few metabolism-mediated drug-drug interaction studies are available in the literature for didanosine, which is not known to be metabolized by CYP450, UGT, or transporter enzymes. The effects of didanosine on the pharmacokinetics of other agents have not been well characterized, and the documented drug interactions are primarily related to altered absorption (e.g., ciprofloxacin, delavirdine, ketoconazole) of co-administered agents, mostly from the use of buffered didanosine dosage forms. The separation of administration times with these agents usually resolves the interactions [43]. On the other hand, the other documented, statistically significant pharmacokinetic interactions (Table 6.7) usually exhibited relatively small magnitudes (~10 %) and had no clear pharmacological basis supporting the interactions. These effects are likely due to the small sample sizes and large variabilities found in the experiments [43] and are unlikely clinically significant.

6.2.3   *Emtricitabine* (Table 6.8)

Little information is available in the literature on drug-drug interactions associated with emtricitabine in humans, which may be due to its lack of pharmacological basis for metabolism-related interactions (Chap. 4). The manufacturer has conducted a number of experiments to determine the effects of emtricitabine on the pharmacokinetics of various co-administered antivirals (famciclovir, indinavir, tenofovir, stavudine, and zidovudine) [44] in healthy volunteers (Table 6.8), and the majority of the findings have reported no observable interactions. Steady-state emtricitabine (200 mg daily) did significantly increase the AUC (13 %) and Cmax (17 %) of zidovudine (300 mg twice daily, $N = 27$), but these effects were minimal and unlikely translated to a significant pharmacodynamic effect. No clear pharmacological basis explained the statistical significant interaction between these two agents.

Table 6.6 Effects of abacavir on the pharmacokinetics of co-administered drugs

Drug	Summary effects on pharmacokinetics	Reference
Limited published studies are available characterizing metabolism-mediated drug-interactions caused by abacavir		

Table 6.7 Effects of didanosine on the pharmacokinetics of co-administered drugs [43]

Drug	Summary effects on pharmacokinetics	Reference
Ciprofloxacin	↓ AUC (26 %), ↓ Cmax (16 %)	FDA document
Delavirdine	↓ AUC (32 %), ↓ Cmax (53 %)	FDA document
Ketoconazole	↓ AUC (14 %), ↓ Cmax (20 %)	FDA document
Nelfinavir	↑ AUC (12 %)	FDA document
Dapsone	No significant change in pharmacokinetic parameters	FDA document
Ranitidine	↓ AUC (16 %)	FDA document
Ritonavir	No significant change in pharmacokinetic parameters	FDA document
Stavudine	No significant change in pharmacokinetic parameters	FDA document
Sulfamethoxazole	↓ AUC (11 %), ↓ Cmax (12 %)	FDA document
Tenofovir	No significant change in pharmacokinetic parameters	FDA document
Trimethoprim	↑ AUC (10 %), ↓ Cmax (22 %)	FDA document
Zidovudine	↓ AUC (10 %), ↓ Cmax (16.5 %)	FDA document

AUC area-under-the curve, *Cmax* maximum concentration

Table 6.8 Effects of emtricitabine on the pharmacokinetics of co-administered drugs [44]

Drug	Summary effects on pharmacokinetics	Reference
Famciclovir	No significant change in pharmacokinetic parameters	FDA document
Indinavir	No significant change in pharmacokinetic parameters	FDA document
Tenofovir	No significant change in pharmacokinetic parameters	FDA document
Stavudine	No significant change in pharmacokinetic parameters	FDA document
Zidovudine	↑ AUC (13 %), ↑ Cmax (17 %)	FDA document

AUC area-under-the curve, *Cmax* maximum concentration

6.2.4 *Lamivudine* (Table 6.9)

A paucity of literature has been published describing the drug-drug interactions associated with lamivudine in humans (Table 6.9). Steady-state lamivudine did not affect the pharmacokinetics of zidovudine in HIV-infected patients ($N = 12$) or interferon alpha in healthy volunteers ($N = 19$) [45]. Despite a significant effect from

Table 6.9 Effects of lamivudine on the pharmacokinetics of co-administered drugs [45]

Drug	Summary effects on pharmacokinetics	Reference
Interferon alpha	No significant change in pharmacokinetic parameters	FDA document
Trimethoprim/sulfamethoxazole	No significant change in pharmacokinetic parameters	FDA document
Zidovudine	No significant change in pharmacokinetic parameters	FDA document

trimethoprim/sulfamethoxazole on the exposure of lamivudine (Chap. 5), lamivu-dine (300 mg every 12 h) did not change the pharmacokinetics of trimethoprim or sulfamethoxazole (160 mg/800 mg daily) in HIV-infected patients under steady-state conditions ($N=14$). These findings are consistent with the lack of pharmaco-logical basis for metabolism-related interactions associated with lamivudine in general (Chap. 4).

6.2.5   *Stavudine* (Table 6.10)

Little information is available in the literature on drug-drug interactions associated with stavudine in humans. In HIV-infected subjects, stavudine (40 mg as single dose or multiple doses) did not alter the pharmacokinetics of didanosine (100 mg every 12 h × 4 days), lamivudine (150 mg as single dose), and nelfinavir (750 mg every 8 h, steady-state conditions) ($N=8–18$) [46] (Table 6.10). These observations are supported by the lack of pharmacological basis for metabolism-related interactions associated with stavudine in general (Chap. 4).

6.2.6   *Tenofovir* (Table 6.11)

Few literature reports have been published describing the drug-drug interactions associated with tenofovir in humans (Table 6.11), and the majority of the available data suggest a lack of significant change in the pharmacokinetics of co-adminis-tered drugs in the presence of tenofovir (Table 6.11) [47–49]. This is consistent with the lack of pharmacological basis for metabolism-related interactions associ-ated with tenofovir in general (Chap. 4) (Table 6.11). Even though tenofovir (300 mg daily) decreased the AUC (25 %) of atazanavir (400 mg daily, $N=33$) and increased the AUC (29 %) of saquinavir (saquinavir/ritonavir, 1000 mg/100 mg twice daily, $N=32$), the mechanisms associated with these significant findings could not be derived from the known metabolic characteristics of the drugs involved. It is also unlikely that the relatively modest changes in atazanavir and

Table 6.10   Effects of stavudine on the pharmacokinetics of co-administered drugs [46]

Drug	Summary effects on pharmacokinetics	Reference
Didanosine	No significant changes in pharmacokinetic parameters	FDA document
Lamivudine	No significant changes in pharmacokinetic parameters	FDA document
Nelfinavir	No significant changes in pharmacokinetic parameters	FDA document

Table 6.11   Effects of tenofovir on the pharmacokinetics of co-administered drugs [47–49]

Drug	Summary effects on pharmacokinetics	Reference
Abacavir	No significant change in pharmacokinetic parameters	FDA document
Atazanavir	↓ AUC (25 %), ↓ Cmax (21 %)	FDA document
Buprenorphine	No significant change in pharmacokinetic parameters	Baker 2010
Didanosine	No change in AUC, ↓ Cmax (20 %)	FDA document
Emtricitabine	No significant change in pharmacokinetic parameters	FDA document
Entecavir	↑ AUC (13 %)	FDA document
Indinavir	No significant change in pharmacokinetic parameters	FDA document
Lamivudine	No change in AUC, ↓ Cmax (24 %)	FDA document
Lopinavir/ritonavir	No significant change in pharmacokinetic parameters	FDA document
Raltegravir	No significant change in pharmacokinetic parameters	Wenning 2008
Saquinavir/ritonavir	↑ AUC (29 %), ↑ Cmax (22 %)	FDA document

AUC area-under-the curve, *Cmax* maximum concentration

saquinavir AUCs would lead to clinically relevant changes in pharmacodynamic effects in the clinic.

6.2.7   *Zidovudine* (Table 6.12)

Little is known of the drug interaction potential of zidovudine in humans (Chap. 4). Despite significant effects by atovaquone, lamivudine, methadone, nelfinavir, and ritonavir on the exposure of zidovudine (Chap. 5), zidovudine did not change the pharmacokinetic characteristics of these co-administered agents (Table 6.12) [50]. Because zidovudine is primarily conjugated by UGT enzymes [16] and also undergoes significant CYP450-mediated oxidation, it can theoretically act as a competitive inhibitor toward co-administered drugs metabolized by these systems. Further data are needed to characterize the interaction potential of zidovudine in the clinic.

6.3   Protease Inhibitors

6.3.1   *Atazanavir* (Table 6.13)

6.3.1.1   Antivirals

The effects of atazanavir on the pharmacokinetics of co-administered NNRTIs and NRTIs have been described in detail in other sections. Please refer to each individual table for details.

The pharmacokinetic interaction between the hepatitis C protease inhibitor, boceprevir, and atazanavir has been characterized in healthy subjects ($N = 39$) [51]. Atazanavir (300 mg daily, boosted by ritonavir 100 mg) did not affect the pharmacokinetics of boceprevir (800 mg three times daily) under steady-state conditions, corresponding with unchanged pharmacodynamic effects. The effects of the interaction between boceprevir (a CYP3A4 substrate) [52] and atazanavir (a CYP3A4 inhibitor) [53] are inconsistent with the known metabolic characteristics of either drug. Because boceprevir is capable of decreasing the exposure of atazanavir (Chap. 5), the co-administration of these agents is not recommended.

When saquinavir (1200 mg daily, $N = 13$) was co-administered with atazanavir (400 mg daily), the AUC and Cmax of saquinavir were increased significantly by 449 % and 339 %, respectively, when compared to saquinavir given alone [54]. Although this combination is not administered clinically, this experiment demonstrated the potent inhibitory effects of atazanavir toward CYP3A4, the primarily enzyme responsible for the metabolism of saquinavir [14].

6.3.1.2   Cardiovascular Agents

The effects of atazanavir on the pharmacokinetics of atenolol, diltiazem, rosuvastatin, and rosiglitazone have been characterized in humans [54, 55]. Atazanavir (400 mg daily) significantly increased the AUC of atenolol (50 mg daily, $N = 19$) or diltiazem (180 mg daily, $N = 28$) by 25 % each, under steady-state conditions in healthy subjects. Atazanavir is known to inhibit a variety of CYP450 enzymes [53], but none of these are known to metabolize atenolol in humans. On the other hand, atazanavir-mediated inhibition of CYP3A4 is likely the mechanism responsible for the observed interaction with diltiazem. Based on these significant pharmacokinetic interactions, the co-administration of these agents is not recommended (Chap. 6), although further investigations are needed to determine if altered pharmacodynamic effects of atenolol and diltiazem are evident.

The effects of atazanavir on the pharmacokinetics of rosuvastatin have been determined in healthy volunteers ($N = 6$) [55]. Atazanavir (boosted by ritonavir) increased the Cmax (600 %) and AUC (213 %) of rosuvastatin (10 mg daily) under steady-state conditions. These changes, however, were not correlated with altered

Table 6.12 Effects of zidovudine on the pharmacokinetics of co-administered drugs [50]

Drug	Summary effects on pharmacokinetics	Reference
Atovaquone	No significant change in pharmacokinetic parameters	FDA document
Lamivudine	No significant change in pharmacokinetic parameters	FDA document
Methadone	No significant change in pharmacokinetic parameters	FDA document
Nelfinavir	No significant change in pharmacokinetic parameters	FDA document
Ritonavir	No significant change in pharmacokinetic parameters	FDA document

Table 6.13 Effects of atazanavir on the pharmacokinetics of co-administered drugs [51, 53, 54]

Drug	Summary effects on pharmacokinetics	Reference
Acetaminophen	No significant changes in pharmacokinetic parameters	FDA document
Boceprevir	No significant changes in pharmacokinetic parameters	Hulskotte 2013
Atenolol	↑ AUC (25 %), ↑ Cmax (34 %)	FDA document
Clarithromycin	↑ AUC (94 %), ↑ Cmax (50 %)	FDA document
Diltiazem	↑ AUC (25 %), ↑ Cmax (98 %)	FDA document
Ethinyl estradiol/norethindrone	↑ AUC (48 %) – ethinyl estradiol ↑ AUC (110 %) – norethindrone	FDA document
Ethinyl estradiol/norgestimate	↓ AUC (19 %) – ethinyl estradiol ↑ AUC (85 %) – 17-deacetyl norgestimate	FDA document
Fluconazole	↑ AUC (8 %)	FDA document
Lamotrigine	No significant changes in pharmacokinetic parameters	Burger 2008
Methadone	No significant changes in pharmacokinetic parameters	FDA document
Omeprazole	↑ AUC (45 %), ↑ Cmax (24 %)	FDA document
Rifabutin	↑ AUC (110 %)	FDA document
Rosiglitazone	↑ AUC (35 %), ↑ Cmax (8 %)	FDA document
Rosuvastatin	↑ AUC (213 %), ↑ Cmax (600 %)	Busti 2008
Saquinavir	↑ AUC (449 %), ↑ Cmax (339 %)	FDA document

AUC area-under-the curve, *Cmax* maximum concentration

rosuvastatin metabolite (N-desmethyl-rosuvastatin) formation, suggesting that the interaction is likely not mediated by the hepatic metabolism (i.e., intrinsic clearance) of rosuvastatin. The significant effects on AUC and Cmax may result in increased toxicity of rosuvastatin, as reported in cases of rhabdomyolysis in subjects receiving the combination [56]. These data suggest that the co-administration of atazanavir and rosuvastatin is contraindicated.

6.3.1.3 Miscellaneous Agents

The effects of steady-state atazanavir (300 mg daily boosted by ritonavir 100 mg) on the pharmacokinetics of the antidiabetic agent rosiglitazone (4 mg as single dose) have been documented in human subjects [54]. Atazanavir increased the AUC (35 %) and Cmax (8 %) of rosiglitazone, an effect likely mediated by the inhibitory effects of atazanavir toward CYP2C9 or CYP2C9, the primary enzymes responsible for the metabolism of rosiglitazone in humans [57]. Given the modest change in the pharmacokinetics of rosiglitazone, clinical monitoring is warranted when the combination is administered.

The effects of atazanavir on the pharmacokinetics of a proton pump inhibitor (omeprazole) have been determined [54]. Atazanavir (400 mg daily, $N = 16$) significantly increased the AUC (45 %) and Cmax (24 %) of omeprazole (40 mg once daily) under steady-state conditions. Unlike the effects of omeprazole on the absorption of atazanavir (reduced solubility of atazanavir in a less acidic environment), the observed interaction is likely mediated by the inhibitory effects of atazanavir toward CYP3A4, an enzyme partially responsible for the oxidation of omeprazole.

Studies investigating the effects of atazanavir on the pharmacokinetics of antimicrobials (clarithromycin, fluconazole, and rifabutin) are available [54]. Atazanavir (400–600 mg daily) significantly increased the AUC (94 % and 110 %, respectively) and Cmax (50 % and 18 %, respectively) of clarithromycin (500 mg twice daily, $N = 21$) and rifabutin (300 mg daily, $N = 3$) under steady-state conditions. On the other hand, the exposure of fluconazole (200 mg daily, $N = 29$) increased only slightly (~8 %) from the co-administration of atazanavir (300 mg daily boosted by ritonavir 100 mg) under steady-state conditions [54]. These data corresponded with reduced exposure of the hydroxylated metabolite of clarithromycin (70 %), supporting the inhibition of CYP3A4 by atazanavir (hence reduced intrinsic clearance of clarithromycin) as the mechanism explaining the interaction. The exposure of 25-O-desacetyl-rifabutin increased significantly in the presence of atazanavir, which may be the results of mixed inhibitory/induction effects of atazanavir toward the various enzymes responsible for the oxidation of rifabutin. On the other hand, the effects of atazanavir on fluconazole exposure are likely too small to be clinically significant, but support the likely inhibition of CYP3A4 as the mechanism for the observed interaction. Overall, due to the significantly increased exposure of both clarithromycin and rifabutin, the co-administration with atazanavir is not recommended. However, fluconazole may be administered with atazanavir due to the lack of bidirectional pharmacokinetic interactions observed with the combination.

The effects of atazanavir on oral contraceptive agents (ethinyl estradiol/norgestimate and ethinyl estradiol/norethindrone) have been characterized [54]. Steady-state atazanavir (400 mg daily, $N = 19$) significantly increased the AUC (48 %) of ethinyl estradiol and norethindrone (110 %, in combination with ethinyl estradiol), whereas steady-state atazanavir (300 mg daily boosted by ritonavir 100 mg) decreased the AUC (19 %) of ethinyl estradiol (19 %, in combination with norgestimate). The inhibitory effects of unboosted atazanavir toward CYP3A4 would likely explain its effects toward ethinyl estradiol (i.e. increased exposure), but the apparent opposite effect from ritonavir-boosted atazanavir toward ethinyl estradiol exposure might be the result of mixed enzyme inhibition/induction complicated by the presence of ritonavir. Failure of contraception would be possible when ethinyl estradiol containing oral contraceptives are administered with atazanavir boosted by ritonavir.

The effects of atazanavir on the pharmacokinetics of lamotrigine in healthy volunteers ($N=21$) have been characterized [58]. Steady-state atazanavir (400 mg daily) had little effect toward the exposure of lamotrigine, whereas atazanavir boosted by ritonavir (300 mg/100 mg daily) slightly decreased the AUC of lamotrigine by 32 %, which corresponded with elevated lamotrigine-2 N-glucuronide to lamotrigine ratio (from 0.45 to 0.71). These findings suggest that atazanavir itself has little effect on the glucuronidation of lamotrigine, whereas atazanavir boosted by ritonavir likely increases the conjugation of lamotrigine (confirmed by increased glucuronide formation), with the induction characteristics of ritonavir (Chap. 4) being the source of the interaction. However, the relatively modest pharmacokinetic changes are unlikely to be translated to significant pharmacodynamic interactions. Patients co-administered lamotrigine and atazanavir (boosted by ritonavir) should be monitored closely for reduced lamotrigine efficacy.

6.3.2 *Darunavir* (Table 6.14)

6.3.2.1 Antivirals

The effects of co-administered NNRTIs, NRTIs, entry inhibitors, and integrase inhibitors on the pharmacokinetics of darunavir have been described in detail in other sections. Please refer to each individual table for details.

The pharmacokinetic interactions between the hepatitis C protease inhibitors (boceprevir, simeprevir, and telaprevir) and darunavir have been characterized in humans [59]. Darunavir (600–800 mg/boosted by ritonavir 100 mg, twice daily) significantly reduced the AUC of both boceprevir (800 mg three times daily, $N=12$) and telaprevir (750 mg three times daily, $N=11$) by 32 % and 35 %, respectively, whereas boceprevir (600 mg boosted with 100 mg ritonavir) extensively increased the exposure (159 %) and Cmax (79 %) of simeprevir (50 mg daily, $N=25$) under steady-state conditions. The apparent interactions between boceprevir, telaprevir (CYP3A4 substrates) [52, 60], and darunavir (a CYP3A4 inhibitor) [61] are inconsistent with the known metabolic characteristics of these drugs, suggesting alternative mechanisms, such as the enzyme induction/inhibition effects of the co-administered pharmacological booster ritonavir, may be involved. The effects of darunavir on the pharmacokinetics of simeprevir are also difficult to explain based on known pharmacokinetic characteristics of either agent. The significant reductions of boceprevir and telaprevir exposure may lead to reduced efficacy of these agents, whereas increased exposure of simeprevir may lead to

Table 6.14 Effects of darunavir (boosted with ritonavir or cobicistat) on the pharmacokinetics of co-administered drugs [59, 62]

Drug	Summary effects on pharmacokinetics	Reference
Atorvastatin	↓ AUC (15 %), ↓ Cmax (44 %)	FDA document
Artemether/lumefantrine	↓ artemether AUC (14 %) ↑ lumefantrine AUC (175 %)	FDA document
Boceprevir	↓ AUC (32 %), ↓ Cmax (25 %)	FDA document
Buprenorphine	No significant changes in pharmacokinetic parameters	FDA document
Carbamazepine	↑ AUC (45 %)	FDA document
Clarithromycin	↑ AUC (57 %), ↑ Cmax (26 %)	FDA document
Digoxin	↑ AUC (36 %)	FDA document
Ethinyl estradiol/norethindrone	↓ AUC (44 %) – ethinyl estradiol ↓ AUC (14 %) – norethindrone	FDA document
Ketoconazole	↑ AUC (212 %), ↑ Cmax (111 %)	FDA document
Methadone	↓ R-methadone AUC (16 %)	FDA document
Omeprazole	↓ AUC (42 %), ↓ Cmax (34 %)	FDA document
Paroxetine	↓ AUC (39 %), ↓ Cmax (36 %)	FDA document
Pravastatin	↑ AUC (81 %), ↑ Cmax (63 %)	FDA document
Rosuvastatin	↑ AUC (48 %), ↑ Cmax (143 %)	Samineni 2012
Sertraline	↓ AUC (49 %), ↓ Cmax (44 %)	FDA document
Simeprevir	↑ AUC (159 %), ↑ Cmax (79 %)	FDA document
Telaprevir	↓ AUC (35 %), ↓ Cmax (36 %)	FDA document
S-Warfarin	↓ AUC (21 %)	FDA document

AUC area-under-the curve, *Cmax* maximum concentration

toxicity. Based on these findings, the co-administration of these agents is contra-indicated in the clinic.

6.3.2.2 Cardiovascular Agents

The effects of darunavir (boosted by ritonavir) on the pharmacokinetics of atorvastatin, digoxin, pravastatin, rosuvastatin, and warfarin have been characterized in humans [59, 62]. Mixed effects on the pharmacokinetics of the HMG-CoA reductase inhibitors are observed, where darunavir (300–600 mg/boosted with ritonavir) significantly reduced the AUC (15 %) and Cmax (44 %) of atorvastatin (40 mg daily, $N=15$), but had opposite effects on the AUC of a single dose pravastatin (81 % increase, $N=14$) and steady-state rosuvastatin (48 % increase, 10 mg daily, $N=12$). These effects are inconsistent with the known metabolic characteristics of these drugs, where darunavir, being a potent inhibitor of CYP3A4 (Chap. 4), should theoretically have increased the exposure of atorvastatin, a CYP3A4 substrate [36], and have little effects toward the exposure of rosuvastatin, a CYP2C9 substrate [63]. It is possible that these contradictory findings may be due to mixed enzyme induction/

inhibition effects from the pharmacological booster ritonavir, which has been used with darunavir in these experiments. Based on these significant pharmacokinetic interactions, the co-administration of darunavir (boosted by ritonavir) with these statins warrants close monitoring of patients.

The effects of steady-state darunavir (400 mg boosted by 100 mg ritonavir) on the pharmacokinetics of a single dose of digoxin (0.4 mg) have been determined. Darunavir significantly increased the AUC of digoxin by 36% ($N=8$), an effect likely mediated by its inhibitory effects toward p-glycoprotein transporters [63] that are responsible for the clearance of digoxin. This mechanistic interaction, however, would have to be verified using in vitro experimental models such as primary cultures of human hepatocytes or the Caco-2-cell permeability assay. Due to the narrow therapeutic index of digoxin, close monitoring for signs of digoxin toxicity is needed in patients given the combination.

The co-administration of darunavir (600 mg boosted by 100 mg ritonavir) has an effect on the pharmacokinetics of a single dose of S-warfarin (10 mg, $N=12$) in humans [59]. The significant reductions in AUC (21%) and Cmax (8%) of warfarin corresponded with elevations of 7-hydroxy-S-warfarin, indicating that enzyme induction of metabolic enzymes responsible for the intrinsic clearance of warfarin is likely the mechanism responsible for the interaction. Because darunavir is not a known inducer of enzymes (Chap. 4), the observed effect may be due to the presence of ritonavir, which is capable of inducing various CYP450 enzymes (e.g., CYP1A2, CYP2C9) that are responsible for warfarin metabolism [64]. The potential for decreased anticoagulation efficacy should be followed closely (via INR monitoring) when darunavir (boosted by ritonavir) is co-administered with warfarin.

6.3.2.3 Analgesics

The effects of darunavir on the pharmacokinetics of buprenorphine and methadone have been characterized [59]. Darunavir (600 mg, boosted by ritonavir 100 mg, twice daily) did not affect the AUC or Cmax of buprenorphine (8–16 mg given with naloxone 2–4 mg, $N=17$) but significantly increased the formation of norbuprenorphine. On the other hand, darunavir/ritonavir modestly decreased the AUC (16%) and Cmax (24%) of R-methadone (55–150 mg daily, $N=16$) under steady-state conditions. Because buprenorphine and methadone are primarily metabolized by CYP3A4 [4, 65], the lack of increase in its exposure by darunavir, a potent CYP3A4 inhibitor (Chap. 4), would indicate that another confounding effect might be present. It is possible that these contradictory findings may be due to mixed enzyme induction/inhibition effects from the pharmacological booster ritonavir, which has been used with darunavir in these experiments. The lack of significant pharmacokinetic interactions with buprenorphine and methadone suggests that the co-administration of these agents with darunavir may be tolerated in the clinic.

6.3.2.4   Miscellaneous Agents

Mixed effects of darunavir (400–600 mg, boosted with 100 mg ritonavir) on the pharmacokinetics artemether/lumefantrine (80 mg/480 mg for 6 doses, $N=15$), carbamazepine (200 mg twice daily, $N=16$), clarithromycin (500 mg twice daily, $N=17$), ethinyl estradiol/norethindrone (1 mcg/1 mg, $N=11$), ketoconazole (200 mg twice daily, $N=15$), omeprazole (40 mg as single dose, $N=12$), paroxetine (20 mg daily, $N=16$), and sertraline (50 mg daily, $N=13$) have been characterized in humans [59]. Darunavir significantly decreased the AUC (16%) of artemether and dihydroartemisinin (metabolite), but increased the AUC (175%) of lumefantrine. Likewise, the exposures of ethinyl estradiol and norethindrone were significantly reduced (by 44% and 14%, respectively) in the presence of darunavir (boosted by ritonavir) under steady-state conditions. These effects are contradictory to the inhibitory effects of darunavir toward CYP3A4, the primary enzyme responsible for the metabolism of these drugs. Again, it is likely that these contradictory findings may be due to mixed enzyme induction/inhibition effects from the pharmacological booster ritonavir, which has been used with darunavir in these experiments.

On the other hand, darunavir (boosted by ritonavir) significantly increased the exposures of carbamazepine (45%), clarithromycin (57%), and ketoconazole (212%), which are known CYP3A4 substrates [6, 66]. The mechanism of interaction may be attributed to the inhibitory effects of darunavir toward CYP3A4 (Chap. 4), but it is not apparent why darunavir would increase the exposure of certain CYP3A4 substrates (e.g., carbamazepine, clarithromycin, ketoconazole) but not others (e.g., artemether/lumefantrine). Significant effects from darunavir on the exposures of certain CYP3A4 substrates suggest that the co-administration should be avoided to minimize the occurrence of drug toxicities.

Darunavir (boosted by ritonavir) significantly decreased the exposure of omeprazole (42%), paroxetine (39%), and sertraline (49%). These findings are more likely attributed to the inductive effects of the co-administered ritonavir toward CYP450 enzymes responsible for the metabolism of these agents, because darunavir is not known to have any inhibitory or induction effects toward CYP2C19 (for omeprazole metabolism) [67], CYP2D6 (for paroxetine metabolism) [68], or CYP2C19 (for sertraline metabolism) [27]. Significantly reduced exposure in the presence of darunavir/ritonavir might translate to decreased efficacy, although pharmacodynamic interactions have not been confirmed in human studies.

6.3.3   *Fosamprenavir* (Table 6.15)

Fosamprenavir is a prodrug that is rapidly hydrolyzed in the gut to form the active drug, amprenavir (Chap. 4). The drug interactions discussed in this chapter pertain to the active moiety.

Table 6.15 Effects of amprenavir (± ritonavir) on the pharmacokinetics of co-administered drugs (unboosted combinations will be designated) [55, 69, 71, 72, 74]

Drug	Summary effects on pharmacokinetics	Reference
Atazanavir	↓ AUC (22 %), ↓ Cmax (24 %) No significant changes in pharmacokinetic parameters – unboosted	FDA document
Atorvastatin	↑ AUC (130 %), ↑ Cmax (304 %)-unboosted ↑ AUC (153 %), ↑ Cmax (184 %)	FDA document
Buprenorphine	No significant changes in pharmacokinetic parameters	Gruber 2012
Clarithromycin	No significant changes in pharmacokinetic parameters – unboosted	FDA document
Esomeprazole	↑ AUC (55 %)-unboosted No significant changes in pharmacokinetic parameters with boosted combination	FDA document
Ethinyl estradiol	↓ AUC (37 %), ↓ Cmax (28 %) No significant changes in pharmacokinetic parameters – unboosted	FDA document
Ketoconazole	↑ AUC (169 %), ↑ Cmax (25 %) ↑ AUC (44 %), ↑ Cmax (19 %) – unboosted	FDA document
Lopinavir/ritonavir	No significant changes in pharmacokinetic parameters – unboosted ↑ AUC (37 %), ↑ Cmax (30 %)	FDA document
R-Methadone	↓ AUC (18 %), ↓ Cmax (21 %)	FDA document
Norethindrone	↓ AUC (34 %), ↓ Cmax (38 %) ↑ AUC (18 %) – unboosted	FDA document
Phenytoin	↓ AUC (22 %), ↓ Cmax (20 %)	FDA document
Paroxetine	↓ AUC (55 %)	van der Lee 2007
Posaconazole	↓ AUC (23 %)	Bruggemann 2010
Rifabutin	No significant changes in pharmacokinetic parameters ↑ AUC (193 %),↑ Cmax (119 %)-unboosted	FDA document
Rosuvastatin	No significant changes in pharmacokinetic parameters	Busti 2008

AUC area-under-the curve, *Cmax* maximum concentration

6.3.3.1   Antivirals

The effects of amprenavir on the pharmacokinetics of NNRTIs, NRTIs, entry inhibitors, and integrase inhibitors have been described in detail in other sections. Please refer to each individual table for details.

The pharmacokinetic interactions between protease inhibitors (atazanavir and lopinavir/ritonavir) and amprenavir (± ritonavir) have been characterized in humans [69]. Boosted amprenavir (700 mg twice daily with 100 mg ritonavir, $N=21$) significantly decreased the AUC (22 %) and Cmax (24 %) of atazanavir (300 mg daily, with 100 mg ritonavir) and increased the AUC (37 %) and Cmax (30 %) of lopinavir/ritonavir

(533 mg/133 mg, $N=18$) under steady-state conditions. Because both atazanavir [53] and lopinavir are substrates of CYP3A4 and amprenavir, a potent inhibitor of the enzyme [70], the findings with lopinavir, but not atazanavir, support these metabolic characteristics. It is again possible that mixed enzyme induction/inhibition effects from the pharmacological booster ritonavir may have confounded the observation. Further experiments are needed to test this hypothesis.

6.3.3.2   Antimicrobials

The effects of amprenavir (± ritonavir) on the pharmacokinetics of antimicrobials (clarithromycin, ketoconazole, posaconazole, rifabutin, and rifampin) have been characterized [69, 71]. Unboosted amprenavir (1200 mg twice daily, $N=12$) did not affect the pharmacokinetics of clarithromycin (500 mg twice daily) under steady-state conditions; this observation is inconsistent with the known inhibitory effects of amprenavir toward CYP3A4 (Chap. 4), the primary enzyme responsible for the metabolism of clarithromycin [6]. These findings, if replicated in larger patient populations, would indicate the suitability of using clarithromycin for the treatment of infection in the presence of unboosted amprenavir.

Both unboosted amprenavir (1200 mg single dose, $N=12$) and boosted amprenavir (700 mg twice daily with 100 mg ritonavir, $N=15$) increased the exposure of ketoconazole in humans [69], an effect likely associated with the inhibition of CYP3A4 by amprenavir. Because the extent of increase in ketoconazole exposure was much greater with boosted amprenavir (169 % vs. 44 %) than with unboosted amprenavir, it may be hypothesized that ritonavir contributed to CYP3A4 inhibition (in addition to the effects of amprenavir), therefore further increasing the concentration of ketoconazole. These findings are in contrast to the effects of boosted amprenavir (700 mg twice daily with 100 mg ritonavir) on reducing the exposure (23 %) of posaconazole (400 mg twice daily) ($N=24$), which may be attributed to the induction properties of the co-administered ritonavir on the metabolism of posaconazole. Based on these findings, the co-administration of amprenavir with ketoconazole is contraindicated (due to large increases in exposure), but posaconazole may be considered due to limited changes in the pharmacokinetics of either agent when administered together (Chap. 5).

Differences in the pharmacokinetic interaction between boosted versus unboosted amprenavir can also be demonstrated with rifabutin [69]. Boosted amprenavir (700 mg twice daily, with 100 mg ritonavir) did not affect the exposure of rifabutin (150 mg every other day, $N=15$), but significantly increased the formation of the 25-O-desacetylrifabutin metabolite. This is in contrast to the effects of unboosted amprenavir (1200 mg twice daily, $N=5$) which significantly increased the exposure (193 %) and Cmax (119 %) of rifabutin (300 mg daily). The effects of unboosted amprenavir are associated with known metabolic properties of amprenavir (a potent CYP3A4 inhibitor) and rifabutin (a CYP3A4 substrate), but the contradictory findings with boosted amprenavir are difficult to explain. The apparent increases in rifabutin metabolite formation would indicate the occurrence of enzyme induction (not known to be a property of amprenavir); thus, these findings may be associated with the confounding enzyme induction effects of the co-administered ritonavir.

6.3.3.3 Miscellaneous Agents

The effects of amprenavir (± ritonavir) on the pharmacokinetics of atorvastatin (10 mg daily, $N = 16$), buprenorphine (stably maintained dose, $N = 11$), esomeprazole (20 mg daily, $N = 25$), ethinyl estradiol/norethindrone (0.035 mg/0.5 mg daily), methadone (70–120 mg daily, $n = 19$), phenytoin (300 mg daily, $N = 13$), paroxetine (20 mg daily, $N = 26$), and rosuvastatin (10 mg daily, $N = 6$) have been determined [55, 69, 72] Amprenavir (boosted or unboosted) increased the AUC (130–153 %) and Cmax (184–304 %) of atorvastatin, an effect likely mediated by the inhibitory effects of amprenavir (by itself or boosted by ritonavir) toward CYP3A4, the primary enzyme responsible for the metabolism of atorvastatin [36] Due to the extensive degree of the interaction, the co-administration of these drugs is not recommended. On the other hand, amprenavir (boosted by ritonavir) had little effect on the exposure of rosuvastatin, which corresponded with little change in the concentration of its metabolite, N-desmethyl-rosuvastatin. These findings may be explained by the lack of modulatory effects of amprenavir toward CYP2C9 (Chap. 4), the primary enzyme responsible for the metabolism of rosuvastatin in humans [73]. These results support the use of rosuvastatin over atorvastatin if a lipid lowering agent is needed in combination with fosamprenavir.

Steady-state amprenavir/ritonavir had little effect on the pharmacokinetics of buprenorphine, which corresponded with little change in adverse events or withdrawal effects from the opioid [74]. This is in contrast to the effects of amprenavir/ritonavir on the pharmacokinetics of R-methadone, where the co-administration resulted in decreased AUC (18 %) and Cmax (21 %) of steady-state methadone. However, pharmacodynamic effects were not characterized in this study. The pharmacokinetic findings are inconsistent with the known metabolism characteristics of these agents, where amprenavir would have theoretically increased the concentrations of both buprenorphine and methadone via CYP3A4 inhibition. The apparent lack of pharmacokinetic interaction with buprenorphine and apparent induction with methadone would suggest that other factors (such as the confounding effects of ritonavir) may have contributed to these findings.

Contrasting effects of boosted versus unboosted amprenavir on the pharmacokinetics of esomeprazole and ethinyl estradiol/norethindrone were observed. Amprenavir (boosted by ritonavir) did not change the pharmacokinetics of esomeprazole, decreased the AUC (37 %) of ethinyl estradiol, and decreased the AUC (34 %) of norethindrone, whereas unboosted amprenavir increased the AUC (55 %) of esomeprazole, did not change the pharmacokinetics of ethinyl estradiol, and increased the AUC (18 %) of norethindrone [69]. These contradictory findings are difficult to be explained by the known metabolic pathways of the interacting drugs, as there is little pharmacological basis for amprenavir to modulate the enzymes known to metabolize esomeprazole or ethinyl estradiol/norgestimate. Likewise, the effects of amprenavir/ritonavir on reducing the exposures of phenytoin (22 %) and paroxetine (55 %) are likely not modulated by amprenavir (not known to be an inducer) but rather the effects of the co-administered ritonavir (known inducer of several CYP450 enzymes).

6.3.4 *Indinavir* [75]/*Nelfinavir [76]/Lopinavir* [77–82]/ *Saquinavir* [83, 84]/*Ritonavir/Tipranavir* [85] (Tables 6.16, 6.17, 6.18, 6.19, and 6.20)

Indinavir, nelfinavir, lopinavir, saquinavir, and tipranavir (± ritonavir) have similar pharmacological characteristics compared to atazanavir, amprenavir, and daruna-vir (i.e., primarily a substrate and inhibitor of CYP3A4 and mixed pharmacologi-cal effects with the boosting agent ritonavir); thus, they would exhibit comparable pharmacokinetic interactions as discussed for these protease inhibitors, with slight variations. See Tables 6.16, 6.17, 6.18, 6.19, and 6.20 for the summaries of phar-macokinetic interactions observed with these agents. Because ritonavir is never administered alone, its interaction effects (when combined as a boosting pharma-cological agent) are presented with the other antiviral agents.

6.4 Fusion Inhibitors

6.4.1 *Enfuvirtide* [86] (Table 6.21)

Few drug-drug interactions are expected to be associated with enfuvirtide because it is not known to be extensively metabolized by the common Phase I (CYP450) or Phase II (UGT) enzymes nor transported by Phase III transporters (Chap. 4). To our knowledge, little information has been reported in the literature.

Table 6.16 Effects of indinavir on the pharmacokinetics of co-administered drugs [75]

Drug	Summary effects on pharmacokinetics	Reference
Clarithromycin	↑ AUC (47%), ↑ Cmax (19%)	FDA document
Ethinyl estradiol	↑ AUC (22%)	FDA document
Methadone	No significant changes in pharmacokinetic parameters	FDA document
Norethindrone	↑ AUC (26%)	FDA document
Rifabutin	↑ AUC (54–173%), ↑ Cmax (29–134%)	FDA document
Ritonavir	↑ AUC (72–96%), ↑ Cmax (19–61%)	FDA document
Saquinavir	↑ AUC (360–500%)	FDA document
Theophylline	No significant changes in pharmacokinetic parameters	FDA document
Trimethoprim/sulfamethoxazole	No significant changes in pharmacokinetic parameters	FDA document

AUC area-under-the curve, *Cmax* maximum concentration

Table 6.17 Effects of nelfinavir on the pharmacokinetics of co-administered drugs [76]

Drug	Summary effects on pharmacokinetics	Reference
Atorvastatin	↑ AUC (74 %), ↑ Cmax (122 %)	FDA document
Azithromycin	↑ AUC (112 %), ↑ Cmax (136 %)	FDA document
Ethinyl estradiol	↓ AUC (47 %), ↓ Cmax (28 %)	FDA document
Indinavir	↑ AUC (51 %)	FDA document
Methadone	↓ AUC (47 %), ↓ Cmax (46 %)	FDA document
Norethindrone	↓ AUC (18 %)	FDA document
Phenytoin	↓ AUC (29 %), ↓ Cmax (21 %)	FDA document
Rifabutin	↑ AUC (83 %), ↑ Cmax (19 %)	FDA document
Ritonavir	No significant changes in pharmacokinetic parameters	FDA document
Simvastatin	↑ AUC (505 %), ↑ Cmax (517 %)	FDA document
Saquinavir	↑ AUC (392 %), ↑ Cmax (179 %)	FDA document

AUC area-under-the curve, *Cmax* maximum concentration

Table 6.18 Effects of lopinavir (± ritonavir) on the pharmacokinetics of co-administered drugs [77–82]

Drug	Summary effects on pharmacokinetics	Reference
Artemether/lumefantrine	↓ artemether AUC (40 %) ↑ lumefantrine AUC (470 %)	Kredo 2016
Atovaquone/proguanil	↓ atovaquone AUC (74 %) ↓ proguanil AUC (38 %)	van Luin 2010
Boceprevir	↓ AUC (45 %), ↓ Cmax (50 %)	FDA document
Bupropion	↓ AUC (57 %)	Hogeland 2007
Buprenorphine	No significant changes in pharmacokinetic parameters	Bruce 2010
Desipramine	No significant changes in pharmacokinetic parameters	FDA document
Ethinyl estradiol	↓ AUC (42 %), ↓ Cmax (41 %)	FDA document
Ketoconazole	↑ AUC (204 %)	FDA document
Lamotrigine	↓ AUC (50 %)	van der lee 2006
Methadone	↓ AUC (53 %), ↓ Cmax (45 %)	FDA document
Phenytoin	↓ AUC (31 %)	Lim 2004
Pravastatin	↑ AUC (33 %), ↑ Cmax (26 %)	FDA document
Rosuvastatin	↑ AUC (108 %), ↑ Cmax (366 %)	FDA document

AUC area-under-the curve, *Cmax* maximum concentration

6.5 Entry Inhibitors

6.5.1 *Maraviroc* [87] (Table 6.22)

Little information, to our knowledge, is published on the effects of maraviroc on the pharmacokinetics of co-administered drugs. Maraviroc did not affect the exposures of ethinyl estradiol/levonorgestrel, lamivudine, midazolam (a marker substrate for

Table 6.19 Effects of saquinavir (±ritonavir) on the pharmacokinetics of co-administered drugs [83, 84]

Effect drug	Summary effects on pharmacokinetics	Reference
Atorvastatin	↑AUC (79%)	Fichtenbaum 2002
Clarithromycin	↑AUC (45%) – unboosted	FDA document
Digoxin	↑AUC (49%)	FDA document
Ketoconazole	↑AUC (168%), ↑Cmax (45%)	FDA document
Methadone	↓AUC (19%)	FDA document
Midazolam	↑AUC (1144%), ↑Cmax (327%)	FDA document
Pravastatin	↓AUC (50%)	Fichtenbaum 2002
Rifabutin	↑AUC (44%) – unboosted	FDA document
Sildenafil	↑AUC (210%) – unboosted	FDA document
Simvastatin	↑AUC (3059%)	Fichtenbaum 2002

AUC area-under-the curve, *Cmax* maximum concentration

Table 6.20 Effects of tipranavir (+ritonavir) on the pharmacokinetics of co-administered drugs [85]

Drug	Summary effects on pharmacokinetics	Reference
Amprenavir/ritonavir	↓ AUC (44%), ↓ Cmax (39%)	FDA document
Atazanavir/ritonavir	↓ AUC (68%), ↓ Cmax (57%)	FDA document
Atorvastatin	↑ AUC (836%), ↑ Cmax (761%)	FDA document
Buprenorphine	No significant changes in pharmacokinetic parameters	FDA document
Carbamazepine	No significant changes in pharmacokinetic parameters	FDA document
Clarithromycin	↑ AUC (19%)	FDA document
Ethinyl estradiol	↓ AUC (48%), ↓ Cmax (48%)	FDA document
Lopinavir/ritonavir	↓ AUC (55%), ↓ Cmax (47%)	FDA document
R-methadone	↓ AUC (48%), ↓ Cmax (46%)	FDA document
Rifabutin	↑ AUC (up to 333%)	FDA document
Rosuvastatin	↑ AUC (26%), ↑ Cmax (123%)	FDA document
Saquinavir/ritonavir	↓ AUC (76%), ↓ Cmax (70%)	FDA document
Tadalafil	↑ AUC (133%)	FDA document

AUC area-under-the curve, *Cmax* maximum concentration

Table 6.21 Effects of enfuvirtide on the pharmacokinetics of co-administered drugs

Effect drug	Summary effects on pharmacokinetics	Reference
Limited published studies are available characterizing metabolism-mediated drug-interactions associated with enfuvirtide in the literature		

CYP3A4) [88], or zidovudine (a marker for UGT) [16], supporting the general lack of metabolism-mediated drug-interactions observed *in vitro* (Chap. 4). On the other hand, maraviroc (300 mg twice daily) significantly reduced the AUC (34%) and Cmax (36%) of amprenavir (from fosamprenavir 700 mg boosted with 100 mg ritonavir), but these significant pharmacokinetic interactions were not associated with altered pharmacodynamic effects [89]. There is little pharmacological basis, from the perspective of metabolic enzymes, for the observed interaction between maraviroc and amprenavir, suggesting that alternative pharmacokinetic processes may be involved. These findings suggest that the co-administration of maraviroc and fosamprenavir/ritonavir should be avoided.

6.6   Integrase Inhibitors

6.6.1   *Dolutegravir* [90] (Table 6.23)

The effects of dolutagravir on metformin, methadone, midazolam, ethinyl estradiol, rilpivirine, and tenofovir have been characterized [90–92]. Confirming the general lack of interaction potential from dolutagravir, it (25–50 mg daily, $N = 10$–16) did not significantly affect the pharmacokinetics of methadone (16–150 mg, steady-state), midazolam (3 mg single dose), ethinyl estradiol (0.035 mg single dose), rilpivirine (25 mg once daily), and tenofovir (300 mg daily). On the other hand, dolutagravir (50 mg once to twice daily, $N = 25$) significantly increased the AUC

Table 6.22 Effects of maraviroc on the pharmacokinetics of co-administered drugs [87]

Drug	Summary effects on pharmacokinetics	Reference
Ethinyl estradiol/levonorgestrel	No significant changes in pharmacokinetic parameters	FDA document
Fosamprenavir/ritonavir	↓ AUC (34 %), ↓ Cmax (36 %)- amprenavir	Vourvahis 2013
Lamivudine	No significant changes in pharmacokinetic parameters	FDA document
Midazolam	No significant changes in pharmacokinetic parameters	FDA document
Zidovudine	No significant changes in pharmacokinetic parameters	FDA document

AUC area-under-the curve, *Cmax* maximum concentration

Table 6.23 Effects of dolutegravir on the pharmacokinetics of co-administered drugs [90–92]

Drug	Summary effects on pharmacokinetics	Reference
Metformin	↑ AUC (145 %), ↑ Cmax (111 %)	Zong 2014 Song 2016
Methadone	No significant changes in pharmacokinetic parameters	FDA document
Midazolam	No significant changes in pharmacokinetic parameters	FDA document
Ethinyl estradiol	No significant changes in pharmacokinetic parameters	FDA document
Rilpivirine	No significant changes in pharmacokinetic parameters	FDA document
Tenofovir	No significant changes in pharmacokinetic parameters	FDA document

AUC area-under-the curve, *Cmax* maximum concentration

(79–145 %) and Cmax (66–111 %) of metformin in a dose-dependent manner in healthy subjects under steady-state conditions [91, 92] without affecting the adverse effects of metformin. The mechanism of interaction has been proposed to be due to organic anion transporter 2 inhibition, although this still requires confirmation in mechanistic experiments ideally conducted in in vitro systems. Due to the extent of interaction observed with metformin, dose adjustment may be warranted, especially in the setting of renal dysfunction.

6.6.2 *Elvitegravir and Raltegravir* [93, 94] (Tables 6.24 and 6.25)

Elvitegravir and raltegravir exhibit similar metabolism characteristics compared to dolutegravir (Chap. 4) and thus have comparable (with slight variations) clinical pharmacokinetic interactions. See Tables 6.24 and 6.25 for the documented pharmacokinetic interactions observed in humans.

Table 6.24 Effects of elvitegravir (± ritonavir) on the pharmacokinetics of co-administered drugs [93]

Drug	Summary effects on pharmacokinetics	Reference
Atazanavir	↓ AUC (21 %)	FDA document
Darunavir	↓ AUC (11 %)	FDA document
Didanosine	↓ AUC (14 %)	FDA document
Rifabutin	No significant changes in pharmacokinetic parameters	FDA document
Rosuvastatin	↑ AUC (38 %), ↑ Cmax (89 %)	FDA document
Tipranavir	↓ AUC (11 %)	FDA document

AUC area-under-the curve, *Cmax* maximum concentration

Table 6.25 Effects of raltegravir on the pharmacokinetics of co-administered drugs [94]

Drug	Summary effects on pharmacokinetics	Reference
Darunavir/ritonavir	No significant changes in pharmacokinetic parameters	FDA document
Etravirine	No significant changes in pharmacokinetic parameters	FDA document
Lamivudine	No significant changes in pharmacokinetic parameters	FDA document
Midazolam	No significant changes in pharmacokinetic parameters	FDA document
Methadone	No significant changes in pharmacokinetic parameters	FDA document
Tenofovir	No significant changes in pharmacokinetic parameters	FDA document

6.7 Summary

The effects of antiviral agents on the pharmacokinetics of co-administered drugs are by and large consistent with the known metabolic characteristics already established from in vitro studies (Chap. 4). The NNRTIs tend to have induction effects, whereas the PIs typically exhibit mixed inhibitory/induction effects toward a host of CYP450 (CYP3A4 being one of the primary targets) and UGT enzymes. As discussed in Chap. 5, the majority of drug-drug interactions reported in the clinical literature on antiretroviral agents have involved NNRTIs or PIs. Moreover, due to mixed induction/inhibition characteristics exhibited by some NNRTIs and PIs, the simple paradigm of one-modulator, one-substrate interaction (as reported in most in vitro drug-interaction experiments) does not always hold true because combination antiviral drugs are usually used. In contrast, the NRTIs, the fusion inhibitor (enfuvirtide), and the entry inhibitor (maraviroc) exhibit reduced drug-drug interaction potential mediated by CYP or UGT enzymes, and clinical data confirm few clinically relevant, metabolism-mediated reactions associated with these substrates. The exception within the NRTI class is zidovudine that exhibits similar metabolic characteristics as the integrase inhibitors (dolutegravir, elvitegravir, and raltegravir); these drugs can potentially act as competitive UGT inhibitors themselves. Similar limitations observed in these clinical pharmacokinetic studies have been discussed in Chap. 5 (small sample sizes, lack of full-complement of pharmacokinetic data, and lack of correlation with pharmacodynamic effects). Future studies should ideally focus on collecting the full spectrum of pharmacokinetic data within the HIV-positive patient population and attempt to draw correlations to pharmacodynamic effects already reported in the literature.

References

1. Guidelines for the use of antiretroviral agents in HIV-1-infected adults and adolescents. 2016. Available at: https://aidsinfo.nih.gov/guidelines/html/1/adult-and-adolescent-treatment-guidelines/0. Accessed 19 June 2016
2. McCance-Katz EF, Moody DE, Morse GD, Friedland G, Pade P, Baker J et al (2006) Interactions between buprenorphine and antiretrovirals. I. The nonnucleoside reverse-transcriptase inhibitors efavirenz and delavirdine. Clin Infect Dis 43(Suppl 4):S224–S234
3. Voorman RL, Maio SM, Hauer MJ, Sanders PE, Payne NA, Ackland MJ (1998) Metabolism of delavirdine, a human immunodeficiency virus type-1 reverse transcriptase inhibitor, by microsomal cytochrome P450 in humans, rats, and other species: probable involvement of CYP2D6 and CYP3A. Drug Metab Dispos 26(7):631–639
4. Kobayashi K, Yamamoto T, Chiba K, Tani M, Shimada N, Ishizaki T et al (1998) Human buprenorphine N-dealkylation is catalyzed by cytochrome P450 3A4. Drug Metab Dispos 26(8):818–821
5. Rescriptor (2012) Prescribing information. Available at: http://www.accessdata.fda.gov/drugsatfda_docs/label/2012/020705s018lbl.pdf. Accessed 19 June 2016

6. Rodrigues AD, Roberts EM, Mulford DJ, Yao Y, Ouellet D (1997) Oxidative metabolism of clarithromycin in the presence of human liver microsomes. Major role for the cytochrome P4503A (CYP3A) subfamily. Drug Metab Dispos 25(5):623–630

7. Borin MT, Cox SR, Herman BD, Carel BJ, Anderson RD, Freimuth WW (1997) Effect of fluconazole on the steady-state pharmacokinetics of delavirdine in human immunodeficiency virus-positive patients. Antimicrob Agents Chemother 41(9):1892–1897

8. Voorman RL, Payne NA, Wienkers LC, Hauer MJ, Sanders PE (2001) Interaction of delavirdine with human liver microsomal cytochrome P450: inhibition of CYP2C9, CYP2C19, and CYP2D6. Drug Metab Dispos 29(1):41–47

9. Borin MT, Chambers JH, Carel BJ, Freimuth WW, Aksentijevich S, Piergies AA (1997) Pharmacokinetic study of the interaction between rifabutin and delavirdine mesylate in HIV-1 infected patients. Antiviral Res 35(1):53–63

10. Borin MT, Chambers JH, Carel BJ, Gagnon S, Freimuth WW (1997) Pharmacokinetic study of the interaction between rifampin and delavirdine mesylate. Clin Pharmacol Ther 61(5):544–553

11. Ferry JJ, Herman BD, Carel BJ, Carlson GF, Batts DH (1998) Pharmacokinetic drug-drug interaction study of delavirdine and indinavir in healthy volunteers. J Acquir Immune Defic Syndr Hum Retrovirol 18(3):252–259

12. Chiba M, Hensleigh M, Nishime JA, Balani SK, Lin JH (1996) Role of cytochrome P450 3A4 in human metabolism of MK-639, a potent human immunodeficiency virus protease inhibitor. Drug Metab Dispos 24(3):307–314

13. Hirani VN, Raucy JL, Lasker JM (2004) Conversion of the HIV protease inhibitor nelfinavir to a bioactive metabolite by human liver CYP2C19. Drug Metab Dispos 32(12):1462–1467

14. Eagling VA, Wiltshire H, Whitcombe IW, Back DJ (2002) CYP3A4-mediated hepatic metabolism of the HIV-1 protease inhibitor saquinavir in vitro. Xenobiotica 32(1):1–17

15. Morse GD, Fischl MA, Shelton MJ, Cox SR, Driver M, DeRemer M et al (1997) Single-dose pharmacokinetics of delavirdine mesylate and didanosine in patients with human immunodeficiency virus infection. Antimicrob Agents Chemother 41(1):169–174

16. Barbier O, Turgeon D, Girard C, Green MD, Tephly TR, Hum DW et al (2000) 3′-azido-3′-deoxythimidine (AZT) is glucuronidated by human UDP-glucuronosyltransferase 2B7 (UGT2B7). Drug Metab Dispos 28(5):497–502

17. Mugundu GM, Hariprasad N, Desai PB (2010) Impact of ritonavir, atazanavir and their combination on the CYP3A4 induction potential of efavirenz in primary human hepatocytes. Drug Metab Lett 4(1):45–50

18. Sustiva (2008) Prescribing information. Available at: http://www.accessdata.fda.gov/drug-satfda_docs/label/2008/020972s030,021360s019lbl.pdf. Accessed 19 June 2016

19. Iribarne C, Berthou F, Carlhant D, Dreano Y, Picart D, Lohezic F et al (1998) Inhibition of methadone and buprenorphine N-dealkylations by three HIV-1 protease inhibitors. Drug Metab Dispos 26(3):257–260

20. Trapnell CB, Klecker RW, Jamis-Dow C, Collins JM (1998) Glucuronidation of 3′-azido-3′-deoxythymidine (zidovudine) by human liver microsomes: relevance to clinical pharmacokinetic interactions with atovaquone, fluconazole, methadone, and valproic acid. Antimicrob Agents Chemother 42(7):1592–1596

21. Gerber JG, Rosenkranz SL, Fichtenbaum CJ, Vega JM, Yang A, Alston BL et al (2005) Effect of efavirenz on the pharmacokinetics of simvastatin, atorvastatin, and pravastatin: results of AIDS Clinical Trials Group 5108 Study. J Acquir Immune Defic Syndr 39(3):307–312

22. Robertson SM, Maldarelli F, Natarajan V, Formentini E, Alfaro RM, Penzak SR (2008) Efavirenz induces CYP2B6-mediated hydroxylation of bupropion in healthy subjects. J Acquir Immune Defic Syndr 49(5):513–519

23. Coles R, Kharasch ED (2008) Stereoselective metabolism of bupropion by cytochrome P4502B6 (CYP2B6) and human liver microsomes. Pharm Res 25(6):1405–1411

24. Ji P, Damle B, Xie J, Unger SE, Grasela DM, Kaul S (2008) Pharmacokinetic interaction between efavirenz and carbamazepine after multiple-dose administration in healthy subjects. J Clin Pharmacol 48(8):948–956

25. Kerr BM, Thummel KE, Wurden CJ, Klein SM, Kroetz DL, Gonzalez FJ et al (1994) Human liver carbamazepine metabolism. Role of CYP3A4 and CYP2C8 in 10,11-epoxide formation. Biochem Pharmacol 47(11):1969–1979
26. Carten ML, Kiser JJ, Kwara A, Mawhinney S, Cu-Uvin S (2012) Pharmacokinetic interactions between the hormonal emergency contraception, levonorgestrel (Plan B), and Efavirenz. Infect Dis Obstet Gynecol 2012:137192
27. Obach RS, Cox LM, Tremaine LM (2005) Sertraline is metabolized by multiple cytochrome P450 enzymes, monoamine oxidases, and glucuronyl transferases in human: an in vitro study. Drug Metab Dispos 33(2):262–270
28. Huang L, Parikh S, Rosenthal PJ, Lizak P, Marzan F, Dorsey G et al (2012) Concomitant efavirenz reduces pharmacokinetic exposure to the antimalarial drug artemether-lumefantrine in healthy volunteers. J Acquir Immune Defic Syndr 61(3):310–316
29. Byakika-Kibwika P, Lamorde M, Mayito J, Nabukeera L, Namakula R, Mayanja-Kizza H et al (2012) Significant pharmacokinetic interactions between artemether/lumefantrine and efavirenz or nevirapine in HIV-infected Ugandan adults. J Antimicrob Chemother 67(9):2213–2221
30. van Luin M, Van der Ende ME, Richter C, Visser M, Faraj D, Van der Ven A et al (2010) Lower atovaquone/proguanil concentrations in patients taking efavirenz, lopinavir/ritonavir or atazanavir/ritonavir. AIDS 24(8):1223–1226
31. la Porte CJ, Sabo JP, Beique L, Cameron DW (2009) Lack of effect of efavirenz on the pharmacokinetics of tipranavir-ritonavir in healthy volunteers. Antimicrob Agents Chemother 53(11):4840–4844
32. Kakuda TN, DeMasi R, van Delft Y, Mohammed P (2013) Pharmacokinetic interaction between etravirine or darunavir/ritonavir and artemether/lumefantrine in healthy volunteers: a two-panel, two-way, two-period, randomized trial. HIV Med 14(7):421–429
33. Intelence (2009) Prescribing information. Available at: http://www.accessdata.fda.gov/drugsatfda_docs/label/2009/022187s002lbl.pdf. Accessed 19 June 2016
34. Yanakakis LJ, Bumpus NN (2012) Biotransformation of the antiretroviral drug etravirine: metabolite identification, reaction phenotyping, and characterization of autoinduction of cytochrome P450-dependent metabolism. Drug Metab Dispos 40(4):803–814
35. Hammond KP, Wolfe P, Burton JR Jr, Predhomme JA, Ellis CM, Ray ML et al (2013) Pharmacokinetic interaction between boceprevir and etravirine in HIV/HCV seronegative volunteers. J Acquir Immune Defic Syndr 62(1):67–73
36. Park JE, Kim KB, Bae SK, Moon BS, Liu KH, Shin JG (2008) Contribution of cytochrome P450 3A4 and 3A5 to the metabolism of atorvastatin. Xenobiotica 38(9):1240–1251
37. Ku HY, Ahn HJ, Seo KA, Kim H, Oh M, Bae SK et al (2008) The contributions of cytochromes P450 3A4 and 3A5 to the metabolism of the phosphodiesterase type 5 inhibitors sildenafil, udenafil, and vardenafil. Drug Metab Dispos 36(6):986–990
38. McCance-Katz EF, Moody DE, Morse GD, Ma Q, Rainey PM (2010) Lack of clinically significant drug interactions between nevirapine and buprenorphine. Am J Addict 19(1):30–37
39. Viramune (2010) Prescribing information. Available at: http://www.accessdata.fda.gov/drugsatfda_docs/label/2010/020933s022,020636s032lbl.pdf. Accessed 19 June 2016
40. Edurant (2015) Prescribing information. Available at: http://www.edurant.com/shared/product/Edurant/EDURANT-PI.pdf. Accessed 19 June 2016
41. Weiss J, Haefeli WE (2013) Potential of the novel antiretroviral drug rilpivirine to modulate the expression and function of drug transporters and drug-metabolising enzymes in vitro. Int J Antimicrob Agents 41(5):484–487
42. McDowell JA, Chittick GE, Ravitch JR, Polk RE, Kerkering TM, Stein DS (1999) Pharmacokinetics of [(14)C]abacavir, a human immunodeficiency virus type 1 (HIV-1) reverse transcriptase inhibitor, administered in a single oral dose to HIV-1-infected adults: a mass balance study. Antimicrob Agents Chemother 43(12):2855–2861
43. Videx (2009) Prescribing information. Available at: http://www.accessdata.fda.gov/drugsatfda_docs/label/2009/020156s044lbl.pdf. Accessed 19 June 2016

44. Emtriva (2012) Prescribing information. Available at: http://www.gilead.com/~/media/files/pdfs/medicines/hiv/emtriva/emtriva_pi.pdf. Accessed 19 June 2016
45. Epivir (2013) Prescribing information. Available at: https://www.viivhealthcare.com/media/32160/us_epivir.pdf. Accessed 19 June 2016
46. Zerit (2008) Prescribing information. Available at: http://www.accessdata.fda.gov/drugsatfda_docs/label/2008/020412s029,020413s020lbl.pdf. Accessed 19 June 2016
47. Viread (2012) Prescribing information. Available at: http://www.accessdata.fda.gov/drugsatfda_docs/label/2012/021356s042,022577s002lbl.pdf. Accessed 19 June 2016
48. Baker J, Rainey PM, Moody DE, Morse GD, Ma Q, McCance-Katz EF (2010) Interactions between buprenorphine and antiretrovirals: nucleos(t)ide reverse transcriptase inhibitors (NRTI) didanosine, lamivudine, and tenofovir. Am J Addict 19(1):17–29
49. Wenning LA, Friedman EJ, Kost JT, Breidinger SA, Stek JE, Lasseter KC et al (2008) Lack of a significant drug interaction between raltegravir and tenofovir. Antimicrob Agents Chemother 52(9):3253–3258
50. Retrovir (2008) Prescribing information. Available at: http://www.accessdata.fda.gov/drugsatfda_docs/label/2008/019910s033lbl.pdf. Accessed 19 June 2016
51. Hulskotte EG, Feng HP, Xuan F, van Zutven MG, Treitel MA, Hughes EA et al (2013) Pharmacokinetic interactions between the hepatitis C virus protease inhibitor boceprevir and ritonavir-boosted HIV-1 protease inhibitors atazanavir, darunavir, and lopinavir. Clin Infect Dis 56(5):718–726
52. Chu X, Cai X, Cui D, Tang C, Ghosal A, Chan G et al (2013) In vitro assessment of drug-drug interaction potential of boceprevir associated with drug metabolizing enzymes and transporters. Drug Metab Dispos 41(3):668–681
53. Zheng J (2002) Clinical pharmacology and biopharmaceutics review (21–567). Available at: http://www.accessdata.fda.gov/drugsatfda_docs/nda/2003/21-567_Reyataz_BioPharmr_P1.pdf. Accessed 6 June 2016
54. Reyataz (2015) Prescribing information. Available at: http://packageinserts.bms.com/pi/pi_reyataz.pdf. Accessed 19 June 2016
55. Busti AJ, Bain AM, Hall RG 2nd, Bedimo RG, Leff RD, Meek C et al (2008) Effects of atazanavir/ritonavir or fosamprenavir/ritonavir on the pharmacokinetics of rosuvastatin. J Cardiovasc Pharmacol 51(6):605–610
56. van der Lee M, Sankatsing R, Schippers E, Vogel M, Fatkenheuer G, van der Ven A et al (2007) Pharmacokinetics and pharmacodynamics of combined use of lopinavir/ritonavir and rosuvastatin in HIV-infected patients. Antivir Ther 12(7):1127–1132
57. Baldwin SJ, Clarke SE, Chenery RJ (1999) Characterization of the cytochrome P450 enzymes involved in the in vitro metabolism of rosiglitazone. Br J Clin Pharmacol 48(3):424–432
58. Burger DM, Huisman A, Van Ewijk N, Neisingh H, Van Uden P, Rongen GA et al (2008) The effect of atazanavir and atazanavir/ritonavir on UDP-glucuronosyltransferase using lamotrigine as a phenotypic probe. Clin Pharmacol Ther 84(6):698–703
59. Prezista (2015) Prescribing information. Available at: https://www.prezista.com/sites/default/files/pdf/us_package_insert.pdf. Accessed 19 June 2016
60. Chapron B, Risler L, Phillips B, Collins C, Thummel K, Shen D (2015) Reversible, time-dependent inhibition of CYP3A-mediated metabolism of midazolam and tacrolimus by telaprevir in human liver microsomes. J Pharm Pharm Sci 18(1):101–111
61. Arya V (2005) Clinical pharmacology and biopharmaceutics review (21–976). Available at: http://www.accessdata.fda.gov/drugsatfda_docs/nda/2006/021976s000_Sprycel_ClinPharmR.pdf. Accessed 6 June 2016
62. Samineni D, Desai PB, Sallans L, Fichtenbaum CJ (2012) Steady-state pharmacokinetic interactions of darunavir/ritonavir with lipid-lowering agent rosuvastatin. J Clin Pharmacol 52(6):922–931
63. Neuvonen PJ (2010) Drug interactions with HMG-CoA reductase inhibitors (statins): the importance of CYP enzymes, transporters and pharmacogenetics. Curr Opin Investig Drugs 11(3):323–332
64. Liu L, Mugundu GM, Kirby BJ, Samineni D, Desai PB, Unadkat JD (2012) Quantification of human hepatocyte cytochrome P450 enzymes and transporters induced by HIV protease inhib-

itors using newly validated LC-MS/MS cocktail assays and RT-PCR. Biopharm Drug Dispos 33(4):207–217

65. Kharasch ED, Hoffer C, Whittington D, Sheffels P (2004) Role of hepatic and intestinal cyto-chrome P450 3A and 2B6 in the metabolism, disposition, and miotic effects of methadone. Clin Pharmacol Ther 76(3):250–269

66. Pearce RE, Lu W, Wang Y, Uetrecht JP, Correia MA, Leeder JS (2008) Pathways of carbam-azepine bioactivation in vitro. III. The role of human cytochrome P450 enzymes in the forma-tion of 2,3-dihydroxycarbamazepine. Drug Metab Dispos 36(8):1637–1649

67. Karam WG, Goldstein JA, Lasker JM, Ghanayem BI (1996) Human CYP2C19 is a major omeprazole 5-hydroxylase, as demonstrated with recombinant cytochrome P450 enzymes. Drug Metab Dispos 24(10):1081–1087

68. Jornil J, Jensen KG, Larsen F, Linnet K (2010) Identification of cytochrome P450 isoforms involved in the metabolism of paroxetine and estimation of their importance for human parox-etine metabolism using a population-based simulator. Drug Metab Dispos 38(3):376–385

69. Lexiva (2009) Prescribing information. Available at: https://www.accessdata.fda.gov/drug-satfda_docs/label/2009/021548s021,022116s005lbl.pdf. Accessed 19 June 2016

70. von Moltke LL, Durol AL, Duan SX, Greenblatt DJ (2000) Potent mechanism-based inhibi-tion of human CYP3A in vitro by amprenavir and ritonavir: comparison with ketoconazole. Eur J Clin Pharmacol 56(3):259–261

71. Bruggemann RJ, van Luin M, Colbers EP, van den Dungen MW, Pharo C, Schouwenberg BJ et al (2010) Effect of posaconazole on the pharmacokinetics of fosamprenavir and vice versa in healthy volunteers. J Antimicrob Chemother 65(10):2188–2194

72. van der Lee MJ, Blenke AA, Rongen GA, Verwey-van Wissen CP, Koopmans PP, Pharo C et al (2007) Interaction study of the combined use of paroxetine and fosamprenavir-ritonavir in healthy subjects. Antimicrob Agents Chemother 51(11):4098–4104

73. Neuvonen PJ, Niemi M, Backman JT (2006) Drug interactions with lipid-lowering drugs: mechanisms and clinical relevance. Clin Pharmacol Ther 80(6):565–581

74. Gruber VA, Rainey PM, Moody DE, Morse GD, Ma Q, Prathikanti S et al (2012) Interactions between buprenorphine and the protease inhibitors darunavir-ritonavir and fosamprenavir-ritonavir. Clin Infect Dis 54(3):414–423

75. Crixivan (2008) Prescribing information. Available at: http://www.accessdata.fda.gov/drug-satfda_docs/label/2008/020685s066lbl.pdf. Accessed 19 June 2016

76. Viracept (2011) Prescribing information. Available at: http://www.accessdata.fda.gov/drug-satfda_docs/label/2011/020778s035,020779s056,021503s017lbl.pdf. Accessed 19 June 2016

77. Kaletra (2013) Prescribing information. Available at: http://www.accessdata.fda.gov/drug-satfda_docs/label/2013/021226s037lbl.pdf. Accessed 19 June 2016

78. Kredo T, Mauff K, Workman L, Van der Walt JS, Wiesner L, Smith PJ et al (2016) The interac-tion between artemether-lumefantrine and lopinavir/ritonavir-based antiretroviral therapy in HIV-1 infected patients. BMC Infect Dis 16:30. doi:10.1186/s12879-016-1345-1 (Published online 2016 Jan 27)

79. Hogeland GW, Swindells S, McNabb JC, Kashuba AD, Yee GC, Lindley CM (2007) Lopinavir/ritonavir reduces bupropion plasma concentrations in healthy subjects. Clin Pharmacol Ther 81(1):69–75

80. Bruce RD, Altice FL, Moody DE, Morse GD, Andrews L, Lin SN et al (2010) Pharmacokinetic interactions between buprenorphine/naloxone and once-daily lopinavir/ritonavir. J Acquir Immune Defic Syndr 54(5):511–514

81. van der Lee MJ, Dawood L, ter Hofstede HJ, de Graaff-Teulen MJ, van Ewijk-Beneken Kolmer EW, Caliskan-Yassen N et al (2006) Lopinavir/ritonavir reduces lamotrigine plasma concen-trations in healthy subjects. Clin Pharmacol Ther 80(2):159–168

82. Lim ML, Min SS, Eron JJ, Bertz RJ, Robinson M, Gaedigk A et al (2004) Coadministration of lopinavir/ritonavir and phenytoin results in two-way drug interaction through cytochrome P-450 induction. J Acquir Immune Defic Syndr 36(5):1034–1040

83. Invirase (2010) Prescribing information. Available at: http://www.accessdata.fda.gov/drug-satfda_docs/label/2010/020628s032,021785s009lbl.pdf. Accessed 19 June 2016

84. Fichtenbaum CJ, Gerber JG, Rosenkranz SL, Segal Y, Aberg JA, Blaschke T et al (2002) Pharmacokinetic interactions between protease inhibitors and statins in HIV seronegative volunteers: ACTG Study A5047. AIDS 16(4):569–577

85. Aptivus (2009) Prescribing information. Available at: http://www.accessdata.fda.gov/drugsatfda_docs/label/2009/021814s006,022292s001lbl.pdf. Accessed 19 June 2016

86. Fuzeon (2011) Prescribing information. Available at: http://hivdb.stanford.edu/pages/linksPages/ENF_PI.pdf. Accessed 19 June 2016

87. Selzentry (2007) Prescribing information. Available at: http://www.accessdata.fda.gov/drugsatfda_docs/label/2007/022128lbl.pdf. Accessed 19 June 2016

88. Gilbertson TA, Liu L, York DA, Bray GA (1998) Dietary fat preferences are inversely correlated with peripheral gustatory fatty acid sensitivity. Ann N Y Acad Sci 855:165–168

89. Vourvahis M, Plotka A, Mendes da Costa L, Fang A, Heera J (2013) Pharmacokinetic interaction between maraviroc and fosamprenavir-ritonavir: an open-label, fixed-sequence study in healthy subjects. Antimicrob Agents Chemother 57(12):6158–6164

90. Tivicay (2013) Prescribing information. Available at: http://www.accessdata.fda.gov/drugsatfda_docs/label/2013/204790lbl.pdf. Accessed 19 June 2016

91. Zong J, Borland J, Jerva F, Wynne B, Choukour M, Song I (2014) The effect of dolutegravir on the pharmacokinetics of metformin in healthy subjects. J Int AIDS Soc 17(4 Suppl 3):19584

92. Song IH, Zong J, Borland J, Jerva F, Wynne B, Zamek-Gliszczynski MJ et al (2016) The effect of dolutegravir on the pharmacokinetics of metformin in healthy subjects. J Acquir Immune Defic Syndr 72(4):400–407

93. Vitekta (2014) Prescribing information. Available at: https://www.accessdata.fda.gov/drugsatfda_docs/label/2014/203093s000lbl.pdf. Accessed 19 June 2016

94. Isentress (2011) Prescribing information. Available at: http://www.accessdata.fda.gov/drugsatfda_docs/label/2011/022145s018lbl.pdf. Accessed 19 June 2016

Chapter 7
Pharmacodynamic Interactions Between Antiretrovirals and Other Agents

Kyle John Wilby, Tony K.L. Kiang, and Mary H.H. Ensom

This chapter will provide an overview of pharmacodynamic drug interactions associated with antiretroviral agents and commonly co-administered agents. By the end of this chapter, the reader will develop an understanding of pharmacodynamic interactions and how they may positively or negatively impact care.

Methodology: Data for this chapter were obtained using the databases PubMed and EMBASE. The following search terms were used in combination: antiretroviral, HIV, nonnucleoside reverse transcriptase inhibitor, nucleoside reverse transcriptase inhibitor, protease inhibitor, entry inhibitor, fusion inhibitor, anti-HIV agents, pharmacodynamic, interaction, synergy, and antagonism. Drug interaction websites were also reviewed to identify interactions not accounted for with the database search.

7.1 Introduction

In contrast to pharmacokinetic interactions, pharmacodynamic interactions are not associated with absorption, distribution, metabolism, or elimination of drugs. Instead, these types of interactions result in additive, antagonistic, or synergistic effects between agents. Additive drug interactions result in increased effects based on the same clinical effects. Antagonistic interactions lead to decreased effects for

K.J. Wilby
College of Pharmacy, Qatar University, Doha, Qatar
e-mail: kjw@qu.edu.qa

T.K.L. Kiang • M.H.H. Ensom (✉)
Faculty of Pharmaceutical Sciences, The University of British Columbia,
Vancouver, BC, Canada
e-mail: tkiang@gmail.com; mary.ensom@ubc.ca

© Springer Science+Business Media Singapore 2016   121
T.K.L. Kiang et al. (eds.), *Pharmacokinetic and Pharmacodynamic Drug
Interactions Associated with Antiretroviral Drugs*,
DOI 10.1007/978-981-10-2113-8_7

both agents. Synergistic interactions result in increased effects to an extent more than only additive between drugs. These types of interactions can affect both efficacy and safety and can also be used for therapeutic purposes if the desired interaction outcomes are known. Alternatively, overlapping toxicities between agents may place patients at a higher risk of experiencing adverse effects.

7.2   Pharmacodynamic Interactions Between Antiretrovirals

Antiretrovirals themselves are prone to pharmacodynamic interactions between drug classes and individual agents. One of the greatest advances in HIV care to date is the use of additive and synergistic interactions to maximize efficacy and antiviral activity as part of highly active antiretroviral therapy (HAART). The rationale for combinations also promotes reduction of drug resistance and allows for maintaining viability of the differing drug classes. The current therapeutic recommendations outlined in Chap. 1 are largely based on both pharmacodynamic and clinical efficacy data factoring considerations regarding efficacy, safety, and drug resistance.

It is likely that many antiretroviral combinations result in synergistic antiviral activity against HIV. While many of these interactions have not been explicitly studied, some data exist that document the extent of synergy between differing drug classes. One study evaluated pharmacodynamic interactions with emtricitabine and tenofovir (recommended nucleoside reverse transcriptase inhibitors [NRTIs]) in combination with all other major classes (nonnucleoside reverse transcriptase inhibitors [NNRTIs], protease inhibitors [PIs], and integrase strand transfer inhibitors [INSTIs]) [1]. The authors infected MT-2 cells with HIV-1 strain IIIb or xxxLAI virus. Effective concentrations that inhibited 50% of viral replication (EC_{50}) were determined for each agent individually and in combination. The pharmacodynamic results were calculated using a combination index (CI) based on data obtained and defined synergy as CI <0.9, additive as 0.9–1.1, and antagonism as >1.1. Findings showed additive to synergistic activity with NNRTIs and PIs. Efavirenz and rilpivirine resulted in CIs of 0.56 and 0.73, respectively. Darunavir, atazanavir, and lopinavir resulted in CIs of 0.77, 0.83, and 0.97, respectively. However, combinations with INSTIs resulted in the strongest synergistic activity with CIs for elvitegravir and raltegravir of 0.47 and 0.52, respectively. When compared, elvitegravir with tenofovir and emtricitabine resulted in more synergistic combination indices compared to rilpivirine ($p=0.03$), atazanavir ($p=0.009$), darunavir ($p=0.002$), and lopinavir ($p=0.002$). No significant difference was noted between elvitegravir and efavirenz combinations. Authors propose an intracellular mechanism for the increased potency and synergistic effect. These findings help to better understand the rationale of antiretroviral combinations and support the use of INSTIs as first-line agents in HIV therapy.

On the other hand, pharmacodynamic interactions between antiretrovirals may result in poor outcomes and make combinations unfit for use. This could be due to additive toxicities or inhibitory mechanisms. From a toxicity perspective, atazanavir should not be co-administered with indinavir due to increased risk of hyperbilirubinemia and jaundice [2]. The NRTIs didanosine and stavudine result in a high incidence of adverse reactions such as neuropathy, pancreatitis, and lactic acidosis and should not be combined. In terms of efficacy, didanosine and tenofovir combinations have resulted in decreased immunological efficacy despite adequate viral suppression. Finally, combinations of stavudine and zidovudine have resulted in antagonism and are not recommended.

An interesting pharmacodynamic interaction was documented between efavirenz and protease inhibitors [3]. In a study with 56 HIV seronegative adults, efavirenz was given on days 1–21 plus amprenavir on days 11–21. A second protease inhibitor (saquinavir, nelfinavir, indinavir, or ritonavir) was given on days 15–21. Findings showed increased total cholesterol (15 mg/dL), low-density lipoprotein cholesterol (LDLc) (10 mg/dL), high-density lipoprotein cholesterol (HDLc) (2.5 mg/dL), triglyceride (16 mg/dL), and glucose (2.3 mg/dL) concentrations during efavirenz and amprenavir after 14 days. Administration and the addition of a second protease inhibitor further increased triglycerides, total- and LDL-cholesterol levels. At a follow-up duration of 42 days (21 days postdiscontinuation of antiretrovirals), total cholesterol, LDLc, HDLc, and insulin all remained persistently elevated. These results show regimens containing both efavirenz and a protease inhibitor which may have undesirable metabolic implications, and patients receiving both medications should be carefully monitored.

7.3 Pharmacodynamic Interactions with Antimalarials

As described in Chap. 3, malaria and HIV are common comorbidities, especially in sub-Saharan Africa. As such, the potential for drug interactions is high. The following examples provide insight into how these interactions may affect both efficacy and safety of therapeutic regimens.

A synergistic efficacy interaction may occur between antiretrovirals and antimalarial agents. An in vitro study found both chloroquine and mefloquine to be synergistic against *Plasmodium falciparum* with the HIV protease inhibitors saquinavir and ritonavir [4]. A similar in vitro finding was also found between chlorquine and indinavir for both chloroquine-sensitive and chloroquine-resistant strains of *Plasmodium falciparum* [5]. This was followed by an in vivo study in a rat model that found synergy with this combination against chloroquine-sensitive and chloroquine-resistant strains of *Plasmodium chabaudi*. The implications of these findings are unclear, but it is possible that protease inhibitors could be new targets as antimalarial agents. However, use should not be encouraged at this time due to increased potential for resistance against HIV if used without other highly active agents.

Overlapping toxicity has also been reported between antiretrovirals and antimalarials. Hepatotoxicity has been reported for amodiaquine and efavirenz in healthy volunteers [6]. Amodiaquine was also associated with prolonged neutropenia in

Ugandan children taking antiretrovirals [6]. While these are only a few examples, it is likely other interactions exist and care should be taken to minimize them through antimalarial selection. This may be especially important for hepatic, cardiac (QT-prolongation), and hematological toxicities as these are likely most applicable for short-term antimalarial use.

7.4 Pharmacodynamic Interactions with Antitubercular Agents

It is unlikely that synergistic or additive interactions exist for efficacy between antiretrovirals and antitubercular drugs. However, antiretroviral therapy may have beneficial effects for the prevention of tuberculosis. A systematic review was conducted to determine the impact of antiretroviral therapy on the incidence of tuberculosis in adults with HIV infection [7]. After identifying and analyzing 11 studies, the authors found antiretroviral therapy is strongly associated with a reduction in tuberculosis incidence across all CD4 count categories. Although the mechanism behind this finding is uncertain, it can be speculated that maintaining immune function is likely what accounts for the positive results.

Some studies have attempted to evaluate the pharmacodynamic effect of drug combinations on viral suppression. One study assessed daily rifapentine and isoniazid therapy in combination with efavirenz [8]. Evaluations were completed at baseline, 2, and 4 weeks of therapy. From a pharmacodynamic perspective, no clinically meaningful reductions in virologic suppression were observed. Seventy-nine of 85 (93%) had undetectable RNA at baseline compared to 71 or 75 (95%) evaluable patients at week 8. It is likely the combination of these agents is safe for at least a 4-week period.

Studies show that raltegravir may minimize the impact of decreased exposure with antitubercular agents. This suggestion is based on dose finding data demonstrating that the antiviral activity of raltegravir is not blunted with doses as low as 100 mg twice daily [6]. This means that antiviral activity could be maintained despite lower overall drug exposure. However, implications of this consideration for patients receiving tuberculosis therapy are unknown.

On the other hand, overlapping toxicities are of great concern for patients taking antiretrovirals and antitubercular agents. Combinations could result in treatment-limiting adverse effects [9]. The most common overlapping toxicity is likely hepatotoxicity, which may occur with any antiretroviral in combination with rifampin, isoniazid, or pyrazinamide and up to 30% of patients could be affected with co-treatment. Gastrointestinal intolerance and drug fever may also present more commonly between all agents. Specific toxicities should also be closely monitored. For example, anemia and neutropenia may occur with zidovudine and isoniazid, peripheral neuropathy with stavudine and isoniazid or ethambutol, rash with nevirapine, other NNRTIs and isoniazid, rifampin, and pyrazinamide, CNS toxicity with efavirenz and isoniazid, bone marrow suppression with zidovudine or efavirenz and rifampin, and ocular effects with didanosine and ethambutol or rifabutin. Therefore, patients co-administered these agents should be followed up regularly and counseled on potential toxicities.

7.5 Pharmacodynamic Interactions with Chemotherapy Agents

Overlapping toxicities likely result in pharmacodynamic interactions between antiretrovirals and chemotherapy agents [10]. Generally, these interactions are considered additive but may at times be synergistic. Specifically, hematological toxicities may occur with the use of agents such as zidovudine. This is especially important for those patients with preexisting bone marrow compromise, as zidovudine is associated with significant hematological toxicity. As such, alternative agents should be considered for these patients if at all possible. Another adverse effect of concern is peripheral neuropathy associated with vinka alkaloids, taxanes, and ifosfamide. This effect could be enhanced by antiretrovirals such as stavudine, didanosine, and zalcitabine. The newer, less toxic agents (lamivudine, emtricitabine, tenofovir) should be considered first line for these patients.

One study assessed pharmacokinetic and pharmacodynamic interactions of HAART with doxorubicin in patients with HIV-associated non-Hodgkin's lymphoma [11]. Patients received a dual NRTI backbone with addition of a protease inhibitor (indinavir, saquinavir, and nelfinavir). No significant effects were found for pharmacokinetic interactions. Doxorubicin area-under-the-curve (AUC) was associated with hematologic toxicity (defined according to WHO grading) when administered as part of the chemotherapy regimen alone. However, this association was not seen when given with HAART. Therefore, increased toxicity between these agents may be due to other pharmacodynamic interactions such as ones that increase intracellular concentrations of doxorubicin. Clinical implications of this finding are not clear, and patients receiving any chemotherapy with antiretrovirals should be closely monitored for development of adverse effects.

7.6 Pharmacodynamic Interactions with Alcohol, Methadone, and Other Recreational Drugs

As described in Chap. 3, use of alcohol, methadone, and other recreational drugs is common with HIV patients. One study assessed both pharmacokinetic and pharmacodynamic interactions associated with efavirenz and alcohol [12]. Ten patients each received a total of 1 g/kg alcohol dissolved in 16 ounces of a fruit-flavored drink at baseline and after initiation of efavirenz (for at least 2 weeks). Neuropsychological responses were measured before and after efavirenz therapy.

Findings showed intoxication and drowsiness ratings were maintained with efavirenz therapy, despite a lower blood alcohol concentration. This finding suggests a pharmacodynamic interaction may occur between these agents that is independent of the pharmacokinetic findings. This finding is not necessarily surprising, as efavirenz is known to have intoxicating effects. As such, patients should be counseled on the potential increased effects of alcohol when taking efavirenz, even at amounts of usual consumption.

Another study attempted to explore the pharmacokinetic implications of using efavirenz and alfentanil [13]. Twelve HIV patients were administered oral efavirenz for a 2-week period. Patients were also administered alfentanil (oral and intravenous) and oral fexofenadine. Efavirenz decreased the magnitude and duration of alfentanil miosis (area-under-the effect curve, AUEC $(0-\infty)$ 4.3 vs. 3.2 mm*hr in control vs. efavirenz groups, respectively). However, no effect was shown on alfentanil pharmacodynamics, as measured by the concentration-miosis relationship.

Douglas Bruce et al. [14] studied interactions between methadone and elvitegravir-cobicistat in 11 HIV-seronegative patients. Subjects were stabilized on methadone for at least 2 weeks. Elvitegravir-cobicistat was administered once daily for 10 days. Pharmacodynamic outcomes were assessed using measures of opioid withdrawal and excess using the objective opioid withdrawal scale (OOWS), the subjective opioid withdrawal scale (SOWS), the clinical opioid withdrawal scale (COWS), and the opioid overdose assessment scale (OOAS). No differences were found on any of these scales during the course of the study and no dosage adjustments were required. This finding suggests no major pharmacodynamic interaction exists between these agents.

McCance-Katz et al. [15] studied pharmacodynamic interactions between the NNRTI delavirdine and either methadone or levo-alpha acetyl methadol (LAAM). Fifteen methadone patients, 10 LAAM patients, and 15 control patients (all HIV-seronegative) were enrolled to complete the study. Delavirdine was administered in all groups for pharmacokinetic and pharmacodynamic analyses. No cognitive deficits, opioid withdrawal symptoms, or adverse symptom complaints were observed throughout the 7-day study period. Although pharmacokinetic analyses showed increased opioid exposure, pharmacodynamic implications cannot be ruled out.

Although the above examples provide conflicting data regarding pharmacodynamic interactions with these agents, patients must be counseled and carefully monitored to ensure adequate outcomes are achieved.

7.7   Pharmacodynamic Interactions with Hepatitis B and C Treatment

Interactions between agents used to treat hepatitis B and C with antiretrovirals are complex, as regimens may have overlapping efficacy and toxicity. Specifically, lamivudine, emtricitabine, and tenofovir have activity against hepatitis B, while entecavir may have activity against HIV [6]. Use of these agents in first-line regimens for either indication may increase risk of developing drug resistance. This is especially true for HIV regimens containing lamivudine without other active hepatitis B agents (NNRTIs and other NRTIs).

Many issues must be considered when discussing hepatitis C therapy, as newer direct-acting agents are being developed and approved for use. Increased nonresponse to antihepatitis C therapy has been shown with co-administration of abacavir with pegylated interferon and ribavirin regimens [16]. Also, combinations of zidovudine with these agents unsurprisingly led to increased hematological toxicity [17]. Other interactions to consider include potential increases in bilirubin with atazanavir and ribavirin and pegylated interferon, as well as neurological toxicity with efavirenz and pegylated interferon [6].

Reviews of drug interactions with new direct-acting antiviral agents with a focus on antiretrovirals identified many pharmacokinetic interactions but failed to identify any meaningful pharmacodynamic interactions [18, 19]. Therefore, pharmacokinetic, rather than pharmacodynamics, data are better suited to guide clinical use at this time.

7.8   Other Pharmacodynamic Interactions

One study assessed interactions between mycophenolate mofetil and an antiretroviral regimen with efavirenz, abacavir, and nelfinavir in 17 HIV patients [20]. Patients were randomized to receive mycophenolate mofetil plus antiretrovirals or antiretrovirals alone after 12 months of receiving the antiretroviral regimen. After 1 year of receiving antiretrovirals, plasma viral load was undetectable at 0 and 120 days. However, viral load increased to detectable levels in three of nine patients in the mycophenolate mofetil group and in all six patients from the antiretroviral group ($p = 0.01$). This finding suggests mycophenolate mofetil may have an additive or synergistic effect in combination with antiretrovirals for inhibition of viral replication.

One study evaluated a synergistic interaction between saquinavir and ritonavir with itraconazole for treatment of *Histoplasma capsulatum* var. *capsulatum* [21]. All procedures were conducted in vitro. Each drug showed antifungal activity during both filamentous and yeast phases. When given together as saquinavir with itraconazole and ritonavir with itraconazole, minimum inhibitory concentrations were significantly decreased for both ($p < 0.05$), suggesting the presence of a synergistic interaction.

Two studies evaluated interactions between antiretrovirals and gliclazide in animal models [22, 23]. Findings from both studies showed efavirenz reduced the activity of gliclazide yet nevirapine did not. Ritonavir and atazanavir also increased the activity of gliclazide in rats. Potential clinical implications of these results should be further studied, especially in light of increased prevalence of diabetes in regions with high HIV prevalence.

A case series reported on the development of serotonin syndrome in patients taking antiretrovirals and fluoxetine [24]. All patients were taking fluoxetine at the time of antiretroviral initiation or switching. In three cases, the addition of ritonavir appeared to result in symptoms of serotonin syndrome (diarrhea, diaphoresis, anxiety, etc.). One case was likely attributed to efavirenz and the remaining case to addition of grapefruit to the patient's diet. In all cases, the presenting symptoms appeared within 1–2 weeks of therapy or diet change. All cases had the symptoms resolve after decreasing the dose of fluoxetine ($N = 2$), discontinuing ritonavir ($N = 1$), discontinuing grapefruit ($N = 1$), or discontinuing other serotonergic agents such as trazodone ($N = 1$). Although all cases were reported with fluoxetine, it is likely that this pharmacodynamic interaction could occur with other serotonergic agents as well.

7.9   Summary

This chapter provided an overview of examples of pharmacodynamic interactions occurring between antiretrovirals and agents from drug classes commonly administered due to comorbidities (See also Table 7.1.). Overwhelmingly, the most common type of interaction noted was the potential for increased toxicity due to overlapping or additive adverse effect profiles. It is therefore important for clinicians to carefully select combinations of medications that minimize this potential and are safe for patient use. Some studies identified potentially synergistic interactions for activity against HIV or other indications, but clinical studies are needed before many of these findings can be implemented into practice. In order to account for additive, synergistic, or antagonistic interactions, clinicians must be vigilant in monitoring patients and suspecting potential drug interactions where appropriate.

Similar limitations observed in these clinical pharmacodynamics studies were discussed in Chaps. 4 and 5 for pharmacokinetic interactions. These include small sample sizes, lack of standardized pharmacodynamics markers and clinical outcomes, and lack of correlation with pharmacokinetic parameters. Furthermore, pharmacodynamics (compared to pharmacokinetic) interactions are less commonly reported in the literature. Future studies should ideally focus on collecting the full spectrum of pharmacodynamics and pharmacokinetic data within the HIV-positive patient population so that appropriate dosage adjustments, if warranted, can be made to optimize outcomes.

Table 7.1 Summary of pharmacodynamic interactions associated with agents commonly administered in combination

Disease State	Agents and references	Interaction type	Example
HIV	All antiretrovirals [1]	Synergy or additive antiviral activity	Emtricitabine and tenofovir result in synergy with integrase inhibitors
	NRTIs [2]	Antagonism	Didanosine and tenofovir decrease immunological efficacy in combination
Malaria	Antiretrovirals, antimalarials [4]	Synergy	*In vitro* activity studies demonstrate synergy between chloroquine and mefloquine with saquinavir and ritonavir
	Antiretrovirals, antimalarials [6]	Additive toxicity	Increased hepatotoxicity occurs with efavirenz and amodiaquine
Tuberculosis	Antiretrovirals, antitubercular agents [9]	Additive toxicity	Increased anemia and neutropenia occur with zidovudine and isoniazid
Cancer	Antiretrovirals, chemotherapy [10]	Additive toxicity	Peripheral neuropathy occurs between vinka alkaloids, taxanes, ifosfamide with stavudine, didanosine, and zalcitabine; hematological toxicity occurs with zidovudine and chemotherapeutic agents
Alcohol intake	Antiretrovirals, alcohol [12]	Additive toxicity	Despite decreased blood alcohol concentrations, efavirenz in combination with alcohol maintains intoxication and drowsiness levels
Opioid dependence	Methadone, alfentanil [13]	Antagonism	Efavirenz decreases the magnitude and duration of alfentanil miosis but has no effect on withdrawal scales
Hepatitis B	Lamivudine, others [6]	Decreased effect	Increased resistance occurs if lamivudine is used as the only active HBV drug within an antiretroviral combination
Hepatitis C	Antiretrovirals and HCV drugs [6, 16]	Antagonism	Decreased antiviral effects are noted with abacavir and pegylated interferon-ribavirin therapy
		Additive toxicity	Increased bilirubin occurs with atazanavir and pegylated interferon and ribavirin

(continued)

Table 7.1 (continued)

Disease State	Agents and references	Interaction type	Example
Transplant	Antiretrovirals, mycophenolate mofetil [20]	Additive / synergistic efficacy	Mycophenolate in combination with efavirenz, nelfinavir, and abacavir result in possible enhanced viral replication inhibition
Diabetes	Antiretrovirals, sulfonylureas [22, 23]	Additive and antagonistic efficacy	Animal studies show efavirenz reduces activity of gliclazide while ritonavir and atazanavir increase activity
Histoplasmosis	Antiretrovirals, antifungals [21]	Synergy	Combinations of itraconazole with saquinavir and ritonavir decrease minimum inhibitory concentrations
Depression	Antiretrovirals, fluoxetine [24]	Additive toxicity	Fluoxetine in combination with ritonavir or efavirenz resulted in serotonin syndrome symptoms in five patients

HBV hepatitis B virus, *HCV* hepatitis C virus, *HIV* human immunodeficiency virus, *NRTIs* nucleoside reverse transcriptase inhibitors

References

1. Kulkarni R, Hluhanich R, McColl DM, Miller MD, White KL (2014) The combined anti-HIV-1 activities of emtricitabine and tenofovir plus the integrase inhibitor elvitegravir or raltegravir show high levels of synergy *In Vitro*. Antimicrob Agents Chemother 58(10):6145–6150
2. Panel on antiretroviral guidelines for adults and adolescents. Guidelines for the use of antiretroviral agents in HIV-1 infected adults and adolescents. Department of Health and Human Services. 2016. Available at http://www.aidsinfo.nih.gov/ContentFiles/AdultandAdolescentGL.pdf. Accessed 15 June 2016
3. Rosenkranz SL, Yarasheski KE, Para MF, Reichman RC, Morse GD (2007) Antiretroviral drug levels and interactions affect lipid, lipoprotein and glucose metabolism in HIV-1 seronegative subjects: a pharmacokinetic-pharmacodynamic analysis. Metab Syndr Relat Disord 5(2):163–173
4. Skinner-Adams TS, Andrews KT, Melville L, McCarthy J, Gardiner DL (2007) Synergistic interactions of the antiretroviral protease inhibitors saquinavir and ritonavir with chloroquine and mefloquine against Plasmodium falciparum in vitro. Antimicrob Agents Chemother 51(2):759–762
5. Li X, He Z, Chen L, Li Y, Li Q, Zhao S et al (2011) Synergy of the antiretroviral protease inhibitor indinavir and chloroquine against malaria parasites in vitro and in vivo. Parasitol Res 109(6):1519–1524
6. Khoo SH, Gibbons S, Seden K, Back DJ. Drug-drug interactions between antiretrovirals and medications used to treat TB, malaria, hepatitis B&C and opioid dependence. Last updated 2009. Available from: http://www.who.int/hiv/topics/treatment/drug_drug_interactions_review.pdf. Accessed 25 May 2016
7. Suthar AB, Lawn SD, del Amo J, Getahun H, Dye C, Sculier D et al (2012) Antiretroviral therapy for prevention of tuberculosis in adults with HIV: a systematic review and meta-analysis. PLoS Med 9(7):e1001270

8. Podany AT, Bao Y, Swindells S, Chaisson RE, Andersen JW, Mwelase T et al (2015) Efavirenz pharmacokinetics and pharmacodynamics in HIV-infected persons receiving rifapentine and isoniazid for tuberculosis prevention. Clin Infect Dis 61(8):1322–1327
9. Semvua HH, Kibiki GS, Kisanga ER, Boeree MJ, Burger DM, Aarnoutse R (2015) Pharmacological interactions between rifampicin and antiretroviral drugs: challenges and research priorities for resource-limited settings. Ther Drug Monit 37(1):22–32
10. Antoniou T, Tseng AL (2005) Interactions between antiretrovirals and antineoplastic drug therapy. Clin Pharmacokinet 44(2):111–145
11. Toffoli G, Corona G, Cattarossi G, Boiocchi M, Di Gennaro G, Tirelli U et al (2004) Effect of highly active antiretroviral therapy (HAART) on pharmacokinetics and pharmacodynamics of doxorubicin in patients with HIV-associated non-Hodgkin's lymphoma. Ann Oncol 15(12):1805–1809
12. McCance-Katz EF, Gruber VA, Beatty G, Lum PJ, Rainey PM (2013) Interactions between alcohol and the antiretroviral medications ritonavir or efavirenz. J Addict Med 7(4):264–270
13. Kharasch ED, Whittington D, Ensign D, Hoffer C, Bedynek PS, Campbell S et al (2012) Mechanism of efavirenz influence on methadone pharmacokinetics and pharmacodynamics. Clin Pharmacol Ther 91(4):673–684
14. Douglas Bruce R, Winkle P, Custodio JM, Wei X, Rhee MS, Kearney BP et al (2013) Investigation of the interactions between methadone and elvitegravir-cobicistat in subjects receiving chronic methadone maintenance. Antimicrob Agents Chemother 57(12):6154–6157
15. McCance-Katz EF, Rainey PM, Smith P, Morse GD, Friedland G, Boyarsky B et al (2006) Drug interactions between opioids and antiretroviral medications: interaction between methadone, LAAM, and delavirdine. Am J Addict 15(1):23–34
16. Bani-Sadr F, Denoeud L, Morand P, Lunel-Fabiani F, Pol S, Cacoub P et al (2007) Early virologic failure in HIV coinfected hepatitis C patients treated with the peginterferon-ribavirin combination does abacavir play a role? J Acquir Immune Defic Syndr 45(1):123–125
17. Mira J, Lopez-Cortez L, Merino D, Arizcorreta-Yarza A, Rivero A, Collado A et al (2007) Predictors of severe hematological toxicity secondary to pegylated interferon plus ribavirin treatment in HIV-HCV coinfected patients. Antivir Ther 12(8):1225–1235
18. Wilby KJ, Greanya ED, Ford JE, Yoshida EM, Partovi N (2012) A review of drug interactions with boceprevir and telaprevir: implications for HIV and transplant patients. Ann Hepatol 11(2):179–185
19. Burgess S, Partovi N, Yoshida EM, Erb SR, Marquez Azalgara V, Hussaini T (2015) Drug interactions with direct-acting antivirals for hepatitis C: implications for HIV and transplant patients. Ann Pharmacother 49(6):674–687
20. Millan O, Brunet M, Martorell J, García F, Vidal E, Rojo I et al (2005) Pharmacokinetics and pharmacodynamics of low dose mycophenolate mofetil in HIV-infected patients treated with abacavir, efavirenz and nelfinavir. Clin Pharmacokinet 44(5):525–538
21. Brilhante RSN, Caetano EP, Riello GB, Guedes GM, Castelo-Branco Dde S et al (2016) Antiretroviral drugs saquinavir and ritonavir reduce inhibitory concentration values of itraconazole against *Histoplasma capsulatum* strains *in vitro*. Braz J Infect Dis 20(2):155–159
22. Mastan SK, Eswar Kumar K (2009) Influence of non-nucleoside reverse transcriptase inhibitors (efavirenz and nevirapine) on the pharmacodynamic activity of gliclazide in animal models. Diabetol Metab Syndr 1(1):15. doi:10.1186/1758-5996-1-15
23. Mastan SK, Eswar Kumar K (2010) Effect of antiretroviral drugs on the pharmacodynamics of gliclazide with respect to glucose-insulin homeostasis in animal models. J Exp Pharmacol 2:1–11
24. DeSilva KE, Le Flore DB, Marston BJ, Rimland D (2001) Serotonin syndrome in HIV-infected individuals receiving antiretroviral therapy and fluoxetine. AIDS 15:1281–1285

Chapter 8
Conclusion and Clinical Decision Algorithm

Tony K.L. Kiang, Kyle John Wilby, and Mary H.H. Ensom

8.1 Conclusion

We have conducted a systematic qualitative review on the pharmacokinetic and pharmacodynamic drug-drug interactions associated with antiretroviral drugs currently recommended by the World Health Organization. The limitations and future directions have been provided in each Chapter Summary. Here, we will present a Clinical Decision Algorithm (modified from a previous algorithm for antimalarials) [1] to help clinicians assess the relevance of identified drug-drug interactions associated with antiretroviral agents.

8.2 Clinical Decision Algorithm: Pharmacokinetics

1. Does the antiviral drug possess pharmacokinetic properties (with respect to absorption, distribution, metabolism, and elimination) that may be subject to and/or mediate pharmacokinetic drug interactions?

    (a) *The majority of the reported literature has focused on metabolism-mediated drug-drug interactions.*

T.K.L. Kiang • M.H.H. Ensom (✉)
Faculty of Pharmaceutical Sciences, The University of British Columbia,
Vancouver, BC, Canada
e-mail: tkiang@gmail.com; mary.ensom@ubc.ca

K.J. Wilby
College of Pharmacy, Qatar University, Doha, Qatar
e-mail: kjw@qu.edu.qa

© Springer Science+Business Media Singapore 2016   133
T.K.L. Kiang et al. (eds.), *Pharmacokinetic and Pharmacodynamic Drug
Interactions Associated with Antiretroviral Drugs*,
DOI 10.1007/978-981-10-2113-8_8

(b) *The metabolism characteristics for each drug have primarily been determined in in vitro reaction phenotyping studies using human liver microsomes which have some inherent limitations (i.e,. does not represent the full complement of all metabolism enzymes available in vivo systems).*

(c) *The identification of antiviral agents based on drug class (i.e., NNRTIs, PIs, NRTIs, fusion inhibitors, entry inhibitors, and integrase inhibitors) can aid the prediction of drug-drug interactions to which each antiretroviral is subjected. For example, the NNRTIs (with some exceptions) are primarily metabolized by CYP3A4 (and subject to modulators of this enzyme), whereas the integrase inhibitors are primarily conjugated by UGT enzymes (and likely subject to interactions mediated by inhibitors/inducers of glucuronidation).*

(d) *The identification of antiviral agents based on drug class (i.e., NNRTIs, PIs, NRTIs, fusion inhibitors, entry inhibitors, and integrase inhibitors) can also aid the prediction of drug-drug interactions mediated by each antiretroviral. For example, the majority of NNRTIs (with some exceptions) are enzyme inducers, the PIs are mixed enzyme inducer/inhibitors, and the NRTIs are relatively inert to drug interactions.*

2. Is there evidence of significant changes in the pharmacokinetics of antiretrovirals or co-administered drugs in humans?

(a) *The evidence should be weighed against limitations of each study (i.e., sample size, variability, target population).*

(b) *The available human data likely only represent a fraction of all possible interactions associated with antiretroviral drugs. However, the data presented in this book may be used as a tool for the prediction of likely (but not yet confirmed) interactions.*

3. Are significant pharmacokinetic interactions related to pharmacodynamic changes in humans?

(a) *This piece of data is the most important for establishing clinical relevance, and yet these pharmacokinetic-pharmacodynamic relationships (efficacy/toxicity) are often not reported in clinical studies. In the absence of such data, a moderately altered pharmacokinetic effect (i.e., <25% change in exposure) is unlikely associated with toxicity or efficacy, given the typically large variabilities observed in human studies.*

8.3 Clinical Decision Algorithm: Pharmacodynamics

1. Does the effector drug possess pharmacodynamic properties (effect on drug or effect on body) that may increase likelihood of drug interactions?

(a) *Clinicians must be conscious of additive, synergistic, and antagonistic properties of drug combinations.*

2. Does the potential combination pair have overlapping toxicities that could subject patients to harm?

   (a) *Overlapping toxicities or exaggerated pharmacological effects must be carefully monitored in patients at risk of these interactions.*
   (b) *Hepatic toxicity is commonly described in the literature for agents typically used in combination with antiretrovirals.*

3. Is there evidence of a clinically significant drug interaction documented in humans?

   (a) *Pharmacodynamic interactions are less commonly reported in the literature, but some evidence does exist.*
   (b) *Clinicians must use their pharmacological and therapeutic knowledge to assist in determination of actual and potential interactions.*

4. If a clinically significant interaction is likely, is there another choice of agent(s) that may be combined instead?

   (a) *Typically, the agents interacting with antiretrovirals should be the ones modified to avoid disruption of viral suppression.*

Reference

1. Kiang TKL, Wilby KJ, Ensom MHH (2015) Clinical pharmacokinetic and pharmacodynamic drug interactions associated with antimalarials. Springer International Publishing AG, Cham. doi:10.1007/978-3-319-10527-7 (eBook). ISBN 978-3-319-10527-7